Sports Nut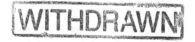 KT-380-264
for Women

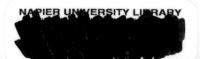

■ Other books of interest from A & C Black

Abdominal Training
by Christopher M. Norris (ISBN 0 7136 4585 7)
This is the definitive guide to developing, safely and effectively, the condition of the trunk muscles – a crucial component of fitness for a variety of sports.

The Complete Guide to Cross Training
by Fiona Hayes (ISBN 0 7136 4993 X)
A comprehensive guide to this increasingly popular area of training, showing precisely how to structure and implement an effective training programme.

The Complete Guide to Exercise in Water
by Debbie Lawrence (ISBN 0 7136 4849 X)
The definitive practical guide for the regular exerciser who wishes to know more about the enormous benefits of training in water.

The Complete Guide to Postnatal Fitness
by Judy DiFiore (ISBN 0 7136 4852 X)
Full of meaningful information and practical advice for the regular exerciser who wishes to do more than just flatten her tummy after having her baby.

The Complete Guide to Sports Nutrition (Second edition)
by Anita Bean (ISBN 0 7136 4388 9)
This highly successful book will show you how improved nutrition can help to enhance performance, boost energy levels, achieve faster and better training gains, and reach higher competitive standards.

The Complete Guide to Stretching
by Christopher M. Norris (ISBN 0 7136 4956 9)
Written by a chartered physiotherapist and sports scientist, this book offers a clearly illustrated guide to stretching, from the principles behind the training to specific recommended exercises.

The Complete Manual of Sports Science
by Wilf Paish (ISBN 0 7136 4854 6)
Sports science is a fast-moving and often bewildering field. This book re-establishes the link between theory and practice by offering a concise and inherently practical guide to the key areas affecting all sports practitioners.

Food for Fitness
by Anita Bean (ISBN 0 7136 4794 9)
A concise sports nutrition guide, an invaluable menu planner and a comprehensive recipe book, all rolled into one. Written to complement *The Complete Guide to Sports Nutrition*.

Sports Nutrition for Women

A practical guide for active women

Edited by Anita Bean
& Peggy Wellington

A & C Black · London

Note
Whilst every effort has been made to ensure that
the content of this book is as technically accurate and as
sound as possible, neither the editors nor the publishers
can accept responsibility for any injury or loss
sustained as a result of the use of this material.

First published 1995 by
A & C Black (Publishers) Ltd
35 Bedford Row, London WC1R 4JH

Reprinted 1996, 1998

ISBN 0 7136 4066 9

A CIP catalogue record for this book
is available from the British Library.

Acknowledgements
Cover photograph courtesy of Jump, Hamburg.
Line diagrams on pages 50, 101, 103 and 125
by Joanna Cameron.

Printed and bound in Great Britain by
Mackays of Chatham

CONTENTS

Contents

FOREWORD

World Champion swimmer **Karen Pickering** (World Short Course Champion 1993, Double Gold Medallist Commonwealth Games 1994 and British record holder) understands exactly how important nutrition is both to performance and health.

'Nutrition is a vital part of my training schedule. I know that I must support my intensive training programme with good nutritional practices, otherwise I cannot train hard and find that I feel constantly exhausted! It's so crucial to me that I have my diet assessed every four months or so, just to ensure that I am getting everything right.

I believe that all females who are involved in an exercise programme should be aware of the importance of sound nutrition. This book is unique in that it provides an ideal opportunity to evaluate common nutrition problems, to assess your own nutrition programme and to update your knowledge about the latest issues related to exercising women. The practical information is invaluable, and written in a simple-to-read style. In conclusion, this book will give most exercisers plenty to think about!'

INTRODUCTION: WOMEN, NUTRITION AND EXERCISE

This book will be invaluable for all women who take exercise and sport seriously. It will enable you to understand the special nutritional demands placed on your body by regular exercise and it will provide an insight into the potential problems that you may encounter as a result of such exercise.

A healthy diet is an essential part of all training programmes, but there are a number of nutritional issues which relate specifically to women, such as bone health, iron deficiency, amenorrhoea and body image. In the following pages, these issues are dealt with in depth by experts in the field of sports nutrition. In addition, active women have special nutritional needs during adolescence, pregnancy and the later years and these are translated into a set of practical guidelines which will help you to cope better with your training programme during these times.

Weight management, body fat and the problems of making weight are in the forefront of the minds of many women; indeed, weight loss or weight control are common motivations for women taking up a particular sport or exercise programme in the first place. However, once the short-term weight goal has been reached (to lose a few pounds, for example), the question often arises: how far should you go? Is a lower than average body-fat level good for health or for sporting performance? Such issues are addressed in chapter 6, which highlights the dangers of inappropriate diets and eating patterns.

There has been some speculation that women with a tendency to eating disorders such as anorexia nervosa and bulimia nervosa are attracted to certain sports and activities which emphasise thinness or low body fat. Aesthetic concerns have become more important than health or performance for many exercising women, with the result that disordered eating patterns are now very common. This has serious health implications for women, resulting in particular in increased risk of amenorrhoea, reduced fertility and bone degeneration. Chapter 8 discusses these dangers

1

and gives practical advice on how to recognise and treat the symptoms.

Each chapter is introduced by an expert in that particular field, and presents the current consensus on that topic. The science has been translated into practical advice and guidelines to enable you to put the information into practice in your own training programme. References and suggestions for further reading are given at the end of each chapter.

Most importantly, you should be able to enjoy your sport *and* enjoy your food. The aim of this book is to help you achieve both – and to keep you in peak health!

NUTRITIONAL NEEDS OF ACTIVE WOMEN

Anita Bean, BSc

> **Anita Bean** BSc received the Exercise Association's 1995 Award for Special Achievement. She has a degree in nutrition and more than 10 years experience advising sportspeople, fitness participants and teams. Author of *The Complete Guide to Sports Nutrition*, Anita has contributed to many national newspapers, magazines (including *Health & Fitness*, *Slimmer* and *Exercise*) and books, and appeared on a number of television programmes. As co-director of P & A Sports Nutrition, she presents courses and seminars nationwide. Anita is a qualified fitness instructor and the 1991 British Bodybuilding Champion.

Regular training places extra nutritional demands on the body, increasing energy production, altering the metabolism of carbohydrate, fat and protein, and affecting body composition. Good nutrition is therefore of supreme importance and can help you both to improve your health and to reach your fitness goals faster. To maximise your performance and get more out of your training programme, you need to fuel your body correctly and provide it with all the essential nutrients. This will help you to increase your energy levels, delay fatigue, train harder and longer and recover more rapidly. This chapter summarises the major nutritional needs of the body during exercise and suggests ways in which you can achieve the right balance of carbohydrate, fat, protein, vitamins and minerals for your particular activity.

Where do I get energy from during training?

Energy for training can be provided by carbohydrate, fat and protein. The proportions used will depend on the type, intensity and duration of your exercise, your fitness level and the amount of carbohydrate in your muscles before exercise.

During anaerobic types of activity (for example, sprinting, weight lifting, kicking, hitting and jumping), carbohydrate alone is used for energy production. During aerobic activities, a mixture of carbohydrate and fat will be used. If carbohydrate is in very short supply – towards the end of a long, hard training session or competition, for example – then protein will be broken down into amino acids to supply the shortfall. This may account for up to 10% of the fuel mixture.

The higher the training intensity, the greater the proportion of carbohydrate used and the lower the proportion of fat. For example, when running at 6 mph, about 60% of the fuel mixture comes from carbohydrate; when walking at 4 mph, about 40% of the fuel mixture comes from carbohydrate and the remainder from fat.

The longer the duration of aerobic activity, the smaller the fuel contribution from carbohydrate and the greater the contribution from fat (and, possibly, protein). Carbohydrate makes a greater contribution at the beginning of an exercise session when stores are higher; as stores gradually become depleted, it provides increasingly less of the total fuel mixture.

Beginners rely more heavily on carbohydrate for fuel at any given exercise intensity. As you become better conditioned and your aerobic fitness improves, fat is more easily broken down and accounts for a higher proportion of the fuel mixture. This is a natural adaptation to training.

What is the best way to fuel my muscles?

For nearly all activities the most important source of energy is carbohydrate. A low intake means low carbohydrate stores and can limit your performance, while an optimal intake can produce a significant improvement in training intensity, duration and performance. Carbohydrate is stored as glycogen in the liver (approximately 100 g) and muscles (approximately 300 g) but, unfortunately, in relatively small amounts. Your glycogen stores can become depleted after 90–180 minutes of endurance activity, after 45–90 minutes of interval training, or after 30–45 minutes of high intensity/anaerobic activity. The consequence of depleted glycogen is fatigue!

Starting exercise with low or sub-optimal glycogen stores leads to:

+ early fatigue
+ reduced training intensity
+ reduced training gains
+ poor performance
+ increased injury risk
+ slower recovery
+ 'burn out' or contribution to overtraining syndrome (if chronic).

How can I speed recovery?

Each time you exercise you use muscle glycogen and reduce your stores, so the aim of your recovery phase is to replenish your glycogen as efficiently as possible before your next workout. You need to consider the following:

+ the amount of carbohydrate in your diet
+ the type of carbohydrate in your diet
+ the timing of carbohydrate intake.

How much carbohydrate?

At a consensus conference on sports nutrition at Lausanne in 1991, scientists recommended that athletes consume at least 60% of energy intake from carbohydrate. This translates into 450 g of carbohydrate for a person consuming 3000 calories a day or 300 g for someone consuming 2000 calories a day. In practice, most active women will need 5–10 g of carbohydrate per kilogram of body weight per day depending on the intensity of their training. The lower end of the range would be suitable for a woman exercising for up to one hour; the upper end would be suitable for an elite athlete exercising for four or more hours a day.

In terms of quantity of food intake, you can get 450 g of carbohydrate from 30 bananas, 12 large potatoes or 10 chocolate bars! Not that such a diet is advisable – this simply gives you an idea of the amount of food that should be eaten. It is more realistic to plan your diet in 50 g portions of carbohydrate. Examples are given below.

Portions of food providing 50 g of carbohydrate

+ three slices of bread or toast
+ one banana sandwich (two slices of bread and one banana)
+ a 6 oz baked potato with 4 oz baked beans
+ 2 oz of breakfast cereal with ½ pint low fat milk
+ 2–3 oz of raisins
+ two or three bananas
+ 1 pint of isotonic sports drink
+ two or three pieces of dried fruit or small cereal bars
+ seven rice cakes
+ 7 oz of cooked pasta
+ 6 oz of cooked rice
+ one bagel
+ four or five oatcakes

Which are the best types of carbohydrate?

There are two main considerations here: first, the nutritional 'package' provided by the carbohydrate source; and second, the speed at which the carbohydrate is absorbed into the bloodstream.

From a nutritional point of view, the best choices are naturally occurring sources of sugars (found in fruit, vegetables and milk) and of complex carbohydrates (found in bread, potatoes, cereals, pasta and grains). This is because they come with a 'package' of other nutrients such as vitamins, minerals, protein and fibre (non-starch polysaccharides).

From a performance point of view, your choice of carbohydrate depends on the timing of intake in relation to your workout. All carbohydrates are broken down into simple sugars and transported as glucose in the bloodstream, and so are equally capable of being taken up by the muscle cells and made into glycogen. As far as glycogen manufacture is concerned, then, it makes no difference whether the carbohydrate comes from packet sugar or wholemeal bread. What you do need to consider is the *speed* at which the carbohydrate is converted into blood glucose and transported to the muscles. The rise in blood glucose levels is indicated by a food's *glycaemic index* (GI): the faster and higher the blood glucose rise, the higher the GI. The GIs of various foods are shown in table 1.

Sometimes it is an advantage to consume high GI carbohydrate – for instance during the first two hours after exercise or towards the end of a long hard workout when glycogen stores are low. Studies have shown that consuming approximately 1 g carbohydrate/kg body weight within the two-hour post-exercise period speeds up glycogen refuelling and therefore speeds recovery time. In contrast, there are times when it is beneficial to consume lower GI carbohydrates in a form in which they are absorbed more slowly over a long period (between workouts; 2–4 hours before a workout). This may be achieved either by selecting moderate and low GI carbohydrates or by combining high GI carbohydrates with low GI carbohydrates, protein or fat. For example, combine rice (high GI) with beans (low GI); baked potato (high GI) with tuna (protein); or bread (high GI) with cheese (protein and fat).

To enable you to choose the right carbohydrates for the right occasion, refer to table 1.

How often should I eat

Eating five or six meals or snacks a day at regularly spaced intervals will help to maximise glycogen storage and energy levels, minimise fat storage, stabilise blood glucose and insulin levels and control blood cholesterol levels. Each time you eat carbohydrate, insulin is produced which allows glucose, amino

Table 1: *The Glycaemic Index of various foods (glucose = 100)*

High		Moderate		Low	
Cereals		**Cereals**		**Pulses**	
White bread	69	Wholemeal pasta	42	Butter beans	36
Wholemeal bread	72	White pasta	50	Baked beans	40
Brown rice	80	Oats	49	Haricot beans	31
White rice	82	Barley	22	Chick peas	36
				Lentils	29
				Kidney beans	29
				Soya beans	15
Breakfast Cereals		**Breakfast cereals**			
Cornflakes	80	Porridge	54		
Muesli	66	All Bran	51		
Shredded Wheat	67				
Weetabix	75				
Fruit		**Fruit**		**Fruit**	
Raisins	64	Grapes	44	Apples	39
Bananas	62	Oranges	40	Cherries	23
				Plums	25
				Apricots	30
				Grapefruit	26
				Peaches	29
Vegetables		**Vegetables**			
Sweetcorn	59	Sweet potatoes	48		
Parsnips	97	Crisps	51		
Potatoes, baked	98	Yam	51		
Carrots	92				
				Dairy products	
				Milk	32
				Yoghurt	36
				Ice cream	36
Other		**Other**		**Other**	
Chocolate biscuits	59	Oatmeal biscuits	54	Fructose	20
Mars Bar	68	Sponge cake	46		
Honey	87				
Sucrose	59				
Glucose	100				
Orange cordial	66				

acids and fatty acids to be removed from the bloodstream and taken up by cells. Therefore, eating moderately and frequently causes a relatively steady insulin release, whereas eating most of your food in one or two large meals causes a more rapid insulin release and less effective glycogen storage. There is also a greater chance of some carbohydrate being converted into fat rather than glycogen.

When should I eat?

Before a workout

Eating a snack meal of low to moderate GI carbohydrate (for example, pasta with chicken or beans) about two to four hours before exercise will help prolong a moderate blood glucose rise. Then, eating 25–50 g of high GI carbohydrate (for example, one or two bananas) just prior to your workout will help increase blood glucose and sustain a higher level for longer in the bloodstream. The optimal timing of this will vary from 5–20 minutes before exercise, depending on the individual.

During a workout

If you are exercising hard for more than one hour, consuming 30–60 g of carbohydrate/hour can help delay fatigue and maintain exercise intensity. The amount depends on your body size (the bigger you are, the more carbohydrate energy you expend) and exercise intensity (the harder you exercise, the more carbohydrate energy you expend). This carbohydrate may be taken in either liquid or solid form. Some people prefer to take a carbohydrate-containing drink, for example an isotonic sports drink or diluted squash, while others prefer to eat carbohydrate in food form, for example bananas and raisins, and to drink water. The choice is yours.

After a workout

It is most important to start refuelling as soon as possible after exercise, as this is when glycogen manufacture is at its most efficient. Studies have shown that eating carbohydrate (1 g/kg

9

body weight) during the first two hours after exercise improves the efficiency of the refuelling mechanism by 5% to 7%. Choose high GI carbohydrates during this period, for example isotonic drinks, bananas, or rice cakes and jam.

How much protein?

Active people need more protein per kilogram of body weight than sedentary people in order to compensate for increased protein breakdown during training and promote new muscle growth and tissue repair. Scientists at the 1991 Lausanne consensus conference on sports nutrition recommended an intake of 1.2–1.7 g/kg body weight each day. In general, the lower end of the range should cover the needs of most endurance/aerobic athletes and the upper end of the range is more appropriate for those involved in strength and power sports. For example, if you weigh 60 kg, aim to consume between 72 g and 102 g of protein per day. In practice, this should represent 12–15% of your total energy intake if you are consuming enough calories to meet your needs (i.e. not dieting). Consult table 2 below to help you work out your daily intake.

Which are the best sources of protein?

You can get protein from many different foods and no one source is necessarily better than another. The usefulness of a particular protein is often measured by its *biological value* (BV), which indicates how closely matched the proportion of amino acids is in relation to the body's requirements. Egg white has a BV of 100, which means that it contains all the essential amino acids which the body requires in closely matched proportions. Therefore, virtually all of the protein provided in the food can be used for making new body proteins.

Other foods with a high BV include milk, cheese, yoghurt, meat, fish, poultry, eggs and soya products.

There are many foods which contain significant amounts of protein but which are short of one or two essential amino acids. These have a low BV and include beans, lentils, peas, bread,

Table 2: The protein content of various foods

Food	Protein (g per portion)
Meat/fish/poultry	
Red meat (4 oz portion)	32
Chicken (6 oz portion)	38
White fish (6 oz portion)	30
Oily fish (6 oz portion)	30
Sausages (2)	15
Mince (4 oz)	25
Tinned tuna (4 oz)	25
Dairy products and eggs	
Milk ($\frac{1}{2}$ pint)	10
Cottage cheese (4 oz)	15
Fromage frais (4 oz)	8
Cheddar cheese (2 oz)	14
Yoghurt (1 carton)	8
Eggs (2)	14
Pulses and nuts	
Kidney beans (8 oz boiled)	15
Baked beans ($\frac{1}{2}$ large tin)	10
Lentils (8 oz boiled)	15
Nuts (2 oz)	13
Cereals	
Bread (2 slices)	6
Pasta (6 oz boiled)	5
Rice (6 oz boiled)	4
Other	
Tofu (4 oz)	9

cereals, grains, nuts and seeds. Eating a mixture of these during the day is equally as good as eating proteins with a high BV. In other words, it is not essential to obtain your protein needs purely from animal sources; a variety of both low and high BV protein foods is a healthy way to meet your requirements.

Why do active women need fat?

It is important to realise that some body fat is absolutely vital. This is called *essential fat* and includes the fat which forms part of your cell membranes, brain tissue, nerve sheaths and bone marrow and which surrounds your organs (heart, liver, kidneys), providing insulation, protection and cushioning against physical damage. In a healthy person, this fat accounts for about 3% of body weight. Women have an additional fat requirement called *sex-specific fat* which is stored mostly in the breasts and around the hips. This fat is involved in oestrogen production and so ensures normal hormonal balance and menstrual function. If it becomes too low, hormonal imbalance and menstrual irregularities result. This fat accounts for a further 5–9% of a woman's body weight.

Fat is also an important energy store, providing 9 calories per gram. It is used during sleep and while sitting, standing and walking as well as during aerobic exercise. This fat comes from adipose tissue distributed all over your body and also from the fat within the muscle cells (this is particularly important during exercise). One kilogram of adipose tissue could supply enough energy for 15–20 hours of exercise. So your fat store is certainly not a redundant depot of unwanted energy!

So, what is a desirable body fat percentage for health? Doctors and physiologists recommend a *minimum* of 5% for men and 10% for women to cover the most basic functions. In practice, a healthy range for men is between 13 and 18%, and for women, between 18 and 25%. Sportspeople are likely to be a little lower. One study of elite athletes found that the men had 4–10% body fat and women 13–18%. However, these are not necessarily recommended levels for health.

How much fat is recommended?

Fat should contribute less than 30% of your total energy intake. This is in line with the recommendations of the Department of Health (less than 33%) and the World Health Organisation (less than 30%) aimed at reducing the risk of heart disease and cancer in the general population. In practice, exercisers who are training to lose weight/fat are usually advised to obtain less than 25% of their energy from fat. For those who have high energy needs (3000 kcal or more), fat should contribute between 25 and 30% of their energy, since it is an energy-dense nutrient and can therefore help to satisfy these needs.

However, you should not reduce your fat intake to below 15–20%, as this can lead to several nutritional problems. If you do, you are unlikely to consume adequate essential fatty acids (linoleic acid and linolenic acid, found in vegetable oils, seeds, nuts and oily fish). These fatty acids make up the structure of cell membranes and are needed to produce hormone-like substances called *prostaglandins* and *leukotrienes* which help to regulate blood clotting and viscosity, the tone of capillary/artery wall muscles, the widening and constriction of blood vessels, inflammatory responses, and your immune system.

The fat-soluble vitamins A, D and E are found only in fat-containing foods, and some fat is needed to enable your body to absorb and transport them. Although you can get vitamin D from ultra-violet light and vitamin A from its precursor, beta-carotene, in brightly coloured fruit and vegetables, getting enough vitamin E can be much more of a problem. It is found in significant quantities only in vegetable oils, seeds, nuts and egg yolk. An important antioxidant that protects our cells from harmful free radical* attack, it is thought to help prevent heart disease, certain cancers and even to retard ageing. It may also help to reduce muscle soreness after hard exercise. So, remember that reducing your fat too far may lead to nutritional and health problems.

What are my vitamin and mineral needs?

Vitamins and minerals play an important role in achieving optimal health and performance. Regular exercise increases the need for many vitamins and minerals, and this can be met from a well planned, balanced diet that also meets your energy requirements. Although individual needs vary, the Department of Health has established a set of *Dietary Reference Values* (DRVs) for each age

* *Free radicals* are atoms or molecules generated during normal energy production which contain an unpaired electron. In large numbers they are capable of damaging cell membranes, DNA, oxidising blood cholesterol and are thought to be responsible for initiating certain cancers and heart disease.

category and sex; this does include a margin of safety. Table 3 shows the *Reference Nutrient Intake* (RNI) for women for most vitamins and minerals. This is the amount judged to be sufficient to cover the needs of 97% of people in that category. In practice, it is more than most people require.

Do I need extra vitamins and minerals?

There is currently no evidence that vitamin and mineral supplements improve performance if you are already meeting your needs from your diet. However, if your diet is low in a particular nutrient, this is likely to have an adverse effect on your health and performance and so supplements may have a temporary benefit. Women who are on restricted diets (for example slimming or vegan diets), or those who have a disordered eating problem, are likely to be lacking in several vitamins or minerals. You should seek professional advice from your GP or a qualified sports nutritionist rather than taking supplements indiscriminately.

Putting the theory into practice is not always easy, especially if you have to travel a lot, eat out or rely on other people to provide your food, and therefore a general multi-vitamin and mineral supplement may be a wise precaution. There is promising and growing evidence that antioxidant nutrients help to reduce the risks of free radical damage and therefore may help protect against cancer, heart disease and premature ageing. They may also help to alleviate muscle soreness resulting from severe exercise.

Do women have any special vitamin or mineral requirements?

In general, women tend to have lower intakes of calcium, iron, riboflavin and folic acid than men. Calcium is important for bone health, and there is evidence that low intakes during childhood and early adulthood may exacerbate other problems common among female exercisers such as low body fat/weight, overtraining, amenorrhoea (absence of periods), psychological stress and eating disorders. A combination of two or more of these factors increases the risk of stress fractures and osteoporosis in

14

later life. This is discussed in greater detail in chapter 3. All active women should aim to consume at least the RNI for calcium. Scientists also recommend that women who are amenorrhoeic should be consuming 1200–1500 mg of calcium daily. Good sources of calcium include milk, cheese, yoghurt, figs, pulses, oranges, sardines, shellfish, white (fortified) bread and flour, nuts and green leafy vegetables.

Iron deficiency anaemia is more common among female exercisers than male. A large proportion of women have depleted iron stores which in itself is not a problem but which may easily develop into iron deficiency anaemia if the body's iron requirements suddenly increase (for example during pregnancy). This is

Table 3: *Reference Nutrient Intakes for vitamins and minerals*

Nutrient	11–15 years	15–18 years	19–50 years	50 + years
Thiamin (mg)	0.7[†]	0.8[†]	0.8[†]	0.8[†]
Riboflavin (mg)	1.1	1.1	1.1	1.1
Niacin (mg)	15[††]	18[††]	17[††]	16[††]
Vitamin B_6	1.0	1.2	1.2	1.2
Vitamin B_{12} (µg)	1.2	1.5	1.5	1.5
Folate (ug)	200	200	200	200
Vitamin C (mg)	35	40	40	40
Vitamin A (µg)	600	600	600	600
Calcium (mg)	800	800	700	700
Iron (mg)	14.8*	14.8*	14.8*	8.7
Zinc (mg)	9	7	7	7
Magnesium (mg)	280	300	270	270

* Insufficient for women with high menstrual losses (iron supplements may be needed)
† Based on energy intake for sedentary women. Actual requirement increases with increasing energy expenditure. The RNI = 0.4 mg/1000 kcal
†† Based on energy intake for sedentary women. Actual requirement increases with increasing energy expenditure. The RNI = 6.6 mg/1000 kcal

usually due to iron loss through menstruation and to generally low iron intake. Many women avoid red meat or eat only very small amounts (one of the richest and most readily absorbed forms of iron), so need to make sure that they obtain enough from other foods such as pulses, wholegrain cereals, fortified breakfast cereals and dark green vegetables. Vitamin C improves iron absorption, so include foods rich in vitamin C (fruit, vegetables or juices) at the same time. Iron supplements are not routinely recommended for active women, but if you suspect that you may be anaemic you should consult your doctor for a blood test and a proper diagnosis. More information about iron deficiency and sports anaemia is presented in chapter 3.

Exercise increases the requirement for riboflavin (vitamin B_{12}), one of the vitamins involved in energy production. Women on low-calorie diets should include plenty of riboflavin-rich foods in their diet such as milk·(this includes low fat milk), cheese, yoghurt, meat and eggs.

Women generally tend to have low folic acid intakes, one of the B vitamins involved in cell division and red blood cell formation. This is particularly important during the first three months of pregnancy, since low intakes may increase the risk of neural tube defects. As a precaution, the Department of Health advises that all women planning a pregnancy take a supplement containing 400 mg folic acid and that they continue to do so up to the twelfth week of pregnancy. This is discussed in more detail in chapter 2.

SPECIAL NUTRITIONAL CONSIDERATIONS FOR CHILDREN AND TEENAGERS

Childhood, puberty and adolescence are periods of rapid growth. During these times, changes in body size, shape and composition take place, especially during the pubescent growth spurt (between 9 and 13 years), and these inevitably increase the requirements for energy and therefore for most nutrients. Children and teenagers involved in sport and exercise are often put under considerable pressure to excel by parents or coaches. They are frequently given well-meaning but misguided advice which can result in various nutrition-related problems such as impaired growth and development, weight problems, eating disorders and dehydration.

How do the nutritional requirements of children and teenagers differ from those of adults?

The nutritional requirements of children and teenagers per kilo of body weight are higher than those of adults because the former are growing quickly and gaining lean body weight. Therefore, their energy intake must be sufficient to support their growth rate as well as their activity level. The table below gives the recommended average energy requirements, but bear in mind that these do not take into account regular exercise or physical training which may amount to an extra 500 or more calories per day. The exact amount will depend on the type, intensity, frequency and duration of training. Also, children are generally less efficient in their movements than adults; in other words, they burn more calories per kg of body weight and may use 20–30% more oxygen per kg body weight to run at the same speed as adults.

The recommendations for carbohydrate (60%), fat (20–30%) and protein (15%) intake are the same for active children and teenagers. In other words, although their total energy intake may be different, the opitimal *proportions* of carbohydrate, fat and protein are no different. A word of caution about carbohydrate foods, though: if the child's requirements are high, do not expect her to obtain all her carbohydrate from bulky, high fibre foods – she may not be able to eat enough. Coaches and parents sometimes forget that children have smaller stomachs, and they apply healthy eating recommendations designed for overweight and sedentary adults to their children with adverse effects. A mixture of bulky, fibre-rich foods (for example wholemeal bread, wholemeal pasta and beans) and less bulky, low fibre foods (for example white bread, sweetened

Table 4: *Estimated average requirements for children and teenagers (Dept. Health, 1991)*

Age	Estimated Average Requirement (kcal/day)
7–10 years	1740
11–14 years	1845
15–18 years	2110

breakfast cereals and confectionery) may be more appropriate for active children and teenagers.

How does their body composition differ from that of adults?

Children and teenagers have a higher body water content, lower bone mineral content and therefore a lower body density than adults. For this reason, the equations normally used for assessing body fat in adults are not suitable for children – they tend to overestimate fatness by 3–6% and underestimate lean body mass. Also, there is a continual fluctuation in fat-free body components. Special equations for estimating body fat from body density measurements and skinfold thickness measurements should therefore be used.

Body composition measurements can be used professionally to monitor changes during a training season and to check that normal development is not impaired. It should be stressed that children should not be put on a standard weight reduction programme. A restrictive diet and/or intense exercise programme to lose fat can seriously harm a child's physical and psychological development.

Should active children and teenagers cut down on fat?

Young, active exercisers do not necessarily have to cut down on fat. It is recommended that they get 20–30% of their energy from fats. Remember that some fat in the diet is vital: fats found in vegetable oils, nuts, seeds and oily fish provide the essential fatty acids which are needed for making prostaglandins (types of hormones) and for the development of nerve and brain tissue. These foods are also good sources of vitamin E, an important antioxidant that helps combat free radicals. Some fat is also needed for absorbing vitamins A, D and E from food.

Fat is also used for energy during rest and exercise. If children eliminate all fatty foods they may not meet their energy requirements.

Perhaps the most important change to encourage is in the *type* of fats eaten. A study carried out at Newcastle University found that about 25% of schoolchildren's fat intake came from meat, meat pies, burgers and sausages, all rich in saturated fats. Children and teenagers should be encouraged to choose lean versions of meat and include some foods that are rich in unsaturated fats.

Are children and teenagers more likely to become dehydrated?

Yes, children have a higher tendency towards heat-related illness than adults. Children do not tolerate extreme temperatures as well as adults because they have a poorer ability to thermoregulate. In other words, their bodies respond differently to exercise: they produce less sweat per sweat gland so do not perspire so readily, and they produce more heat but are less able to transfer this heat from the muscles to the skin. The smaller the child, the greater this excess heat production.

During exercise, children experience a faster rise in their body's core temperature and so are more easily dehydrated than adults. The problem is that children do not instinctively drink enough to replace their fluid losses and often do not recognise the symptoms of dehydration. Since they also acclimatise more slowly to heat, they need to reduce their training intensity for a while and then to build it up again gradually.

Given that children do not recognise dehydration or voluntarily drink enough, it is important that the drink be highly palatable. Water is not so readily drunk and often quenches the immediate thirst sensation before enough has been drunk to rehydrate the body. Flavoured drinks are more appealing. Diluted squash (squash to water ratio of 1:4 to 1:6), diluted fruit juice (between 1:1 and 1:2) or a commercial isotonic/hypotonic sports drink will encourage the child to drink more and also help her to replace fluids faster (*see* also chapter 9 on competition preparation).

Should children and teenagers be encouraged to lose weight?

Embarking on any restrictive diet or on an excessive exercise programme with the aim of losing weight can be dangerous during childhood or adolescence. It can harm physical development and lead to long-term psychological problems. Low calorie or low fat diets are unlikely to support growth and often result in low intakes of protein, iron, calcium and vitamins. Unfortunately, many teenage girls are overly concerned about their appearance and weight and restrict their food intake in an attempt to change their body shape. This can often set the stage for disordered eating patterns and eating disorders later on (*see* chapter 8 on body image).

If a genuine weight problem exists, or if a child is required to make a weight class for competition, then professional help should be obtained from a qualified sports nutritionist.

The combination of chronic food restriction and high energy demands can lead to:

+ glycogen depletion and fatigue
+ lowered nutritional status
+ reduced immune function
+ increased susceptibility to infection and illness
+ hormonal disturbances
+ menstrual irregularities
+ reduced bone density
+ eating disorders.

Should children and teenagers consume more calcium?

Calcium is particularly important for the proper development of the skeleton. Between 85 and 90% of peak bone mass is achieved by the age of 20, and approximately 45% is gained during puberty. The reference nutrient intake (RNI) for girls aged 11–18 years is 800 mg, slightly more than that for adult women, to take into account the increasing bone mass. Results from the Department of Health's survey of schoolchildren's diets in 1989 reveal that girls of 14 and 15 years consumed an average of 692 mg of calcium per day: this may result in a lower peak bone mass and a greater risk of osteoporosis. However, many factors affect bone mass and bone mineral density, including diet, exercise and genetics.

One study has found that children with a higher than average milk (therefore calcium) consumption had a higher calcium retention and bone mineral density than children with a lower intake.

A recent study carried out at the Royal National Hospital in

Bath found a direct link between body weight, bone mineral content and bone mineral density in children aged five, 10 and 21 years. Therefore, growth rate appears to be an important factor determining adult bone mass. This is another good reason why children should not embark on diets or restrict their food intake to lose weight.

Do children and teenagers need extra iron?

The RNI for iron for girls aged 11–18 years is 14.8 mg. During this growth period, extra iron is needed because of the expansion of blood volume and increased tissue mass associated with growth. The onset of menstruation increases iron loss and therefore increases iron requirements. Many teenage girls are at high risk of iron deficiency anaemia due to poor eating habits (for example, dieting, vegetarianism, insufficient iron-rich foods). One study on girls with mild anaemia (haemoglobin < 12 g/dl) showed that they had a lower aerobic capacity than those with normal haemoglobin levels. Good sources of iron include red meat, offal, green leafy vegetables, fortified breakfast cereals and pulses. Vitamin C enhances its absorption. For more information on this topic, refer to chapter 3, *Iron and Sports Anaemia*.

SPECIAL NUTRITIONAL CONSIDERATIONS FOR THE OLDER ATHLETE

More and more women are taking up or continuing exercise programmes and sports in their later years. Certainly, age is no barrier to exercise and fitness. However, as we get older a number of physiological and functional changes take place and some of these can have a bearing on nutritional status.

Do women go into functional decline?

Normally, the ageing process is accompanied by a number of physiological changes. These include:

- a reduction in lean mass of up to 20–30%, with a selective loss of fast-twitch (Type II) muscle fibres
- a reduction in muscle strength
- a reduction in aerobic capacity (up to 30%)
- a reduction in growth hormone production, leading to reduced lean mass
- a reduction in basal metabolic rate (around 10%), and therefore a reduction in calorie requirements
- a reduced immune function and increased susceptibility to infection
- a reduction in flexibility (up to 30%).

However, none of these changes are inevitable, and they can be prevented – or the risk of them drastically reduced – by regular exercise. Lean body tissue can be maintained through appropriate strength training and this maintains the basal metabolic rate. Getting older does not mean that your metabolism automatically slows; changes are related to your total body mass and your lean tissue mass. So most of the functional changes associated with ageing are due to a decrease in activity.

Are older exercisers more prone to dehydration?

Studies have shown that, due to age-related changes in the skin, skin blood flow is reduced in older exercisers. As skin blood flow allows heat to be removed by convection from the body core to the skin, sweating ability may arguably be slightly impaired with the result that heat is less easily dissipated. Thirst sensation may be impaired in some people, and this may exacerbate dehydration.

However, older athletes are equally capable of acclimatising to heat as young athletes. There is a small reduction in thermoregulation, but this is unlikely to impair your performance provided you drink enough fluid (*see* chapter 9 on competition preparation).

Do older exercisers need extra calcium?

It is important to maintain an adequate calcium intake after peak bone mass has been achieved (between 30–40 years), but taking extra calcium from food or supplements will not prevent bone loss or *osteoporosis*. There is some evidence that the age-related loss of bone mass can be slowed down by regular weight-bearing or strength exercise and/or hormone replacement. However, the value of extra calcium is doubtful. Some researchers suggest it may help reduce bone loss, but the Department of Health says that there is not enough evidence to justify increasing the calcium RNI of older women.

Do older exercisers need extra vitamins?

Antioxidants may help to prevent or delay some of the signs of premature ageing. At the moment this evidence comes from studies on laboratory animals, but research underway at the Human Nutrition Research Centre on Ageing at Boston is looking promising.

Antioxidants help to neutralise free radicals. Beta-carotene, vitamin C and vitamin E are perhaps the most well known and well researched antioxidants, but there are dozens of other natural substances in food (for example flavanoids and carotenoids) as well as a number of minerals (for example zinc and selenium) which also have antioxidant properties.

Hard exercise can deplete the body's antioxidant stores if you don't step up your intake. In a recent study, runners were given either an antioxidant supplement or a placebo pill. After six weeks, those who had taken the antioxidant exhibited less free radical damage than those who took the placebo.

It is thought that antioxidants may play an important role in protecting muscle fibres from free radical damage during exercise and reducing post-exercise soreness. At the University of Birmingham, researchers gave volunteers supplements of vitamin C and vitamin E before and after performing one hour of stepping using the same lead leg. They found that those who had taken the vitamin C supplements experienced less muscle damage and recovery was quicker. It was suggested that this was due to its antioxidant properties which helped to protect the muscle cell membranes.

Beta-carotene (per 100 g/3.5 oz)
* Suggested optimal intake is 15–25 mg/day
+ Carrots (boiled)   7.6 mg
+ Red peppers (raw)   3.8 mg
+ Spinach (boiled)   3.8 mg
+ Spring greens (boiled)   2.2 mg
+ Sweet potatoes (boiled)   4.0 mg
+ Mango   1.8 mg
+ Cantaloupe melon   1.0 mg
+ Dried apricots   0.7 mg

Vitamin C (per 100 g/3.5 oz)
* Suggested optimal intake is 100–150 mg/day
+ Blackcurrants   200 mg
+ Strawberries   77 mg
+ Oranges   54 mg
+ Tomatoes   17 mg
+ Broccoli (boiled)   44 mg
+ Green peppers (raw)   120 mg
+ Baked potatoes   14 mg

Vitamin E
* Suggested optimal intake is 50–80 mg/day
+ Sunflower oil   49 mg
+ Safflower oil   40 mg
+ Olive oil   5 mg
+ Sunflower seeds   38 mg
+ Almonds   24 mg
+ Peanuts (plain)   10 mg
+ Peanut butter   5 mg

---

* In the UK there are no recommended amounts set for any of the anti-oxidants except vitamin C (40 mg). Several scientists, including Professor Anthony Diplock from the University of London at Guys Hospital, believe that the UK and US recommended intakes are too low, and Diplock has proposed optimal intakes which would give greater protection from disease. For beta-carotene, the optimal level would be 15–25 mg; for vitamin E, 50–80 mg; and for vitamin C 100–150 mg – all of which are considerably greater than current average intakes.

Which foods are good sources of antioxidants?

Fruit and vegetables contain many of the antioxidant nutrients. The World Health Organisation recommends five or more portions of fruit and vegetables a day – that's about 400 g. At the moment, British people on average eat only 250 g. *Nuts, seeds and their oils* are the richest sources of vitamin E. More evidence is accumulating that *red wine* may help protect against free radical damage, probably due to its protective effect on LDL cholesterol from oxidation. Red wine drinking may explain the 'French paradox', the question of why the French have such a low rate of heart disease despite their high fat diet and high smoking rate. Red wine contains flavenoids from the red grape skins.

Scientists say that it would be difficult to obtain the appropriate levels of vitamin E and beta-carotene from diet alone, so supplements may be the answer. Others are more cautious in making recommendations and go along with the World Health Organisation's emphasis on fruit and vegetable intake.

SUMMARY

- *Carbohydrate* is the most important source of energy for exercise: a low intake can reduce performance and increase fatigue, while an optimal intake can have a significant improvement on training gains, recovery and performance.
- It is recommended that carbohydrates make up at least 60% of the total energy intake.
- Carbohydrate foods which contain a 'package' of other nutrients should form the majority of your intake, but sugars can also play a valuable role.
- It is important to consider the glycaemic index (GI) of the carbohydrate source: high GI carbohydrates are most beneficial consumed immediately prior to exercise, during exercise lasting more than one hour, and within the two-hour period after exercise.
- Your protein requirements are higher than those of sedentary women. An intake of between 1.2 g and 1.7 g per kg body weight per day is recommended to cover the needs of most exercisers (12–15% total energy).

♦ Fat should supply between 20 and 30% of your energy intake.
♦ Very low fat intakes should be avoided: fat is needed for cell membranes, for protecting your organs, and for ensuring normal hormonal balance – they are a source of essential fatty acids, fat soluble vitamins and energy.
♦ Vitamin and mineral requirements are generally satisfied by a well-planned and balanced diet. Higher intakes do not necessarily improve performance or health, although low intakes can have an adverse effect.
♦ Active women should pay special attention to calcium, iron, riboflavin and folic acid intakes.

PRACTICAL POINTS

♦ For optimal performance, aim for 4-5 g of carbohydrate/kg/day if you do less than one hour of exercise a day; 5–6 g/kg/day (1 hour/day); 6–7 g/kg/day (1–2 hours/day); 7–8 g/kg/day (2–4 hours/day) or 8–10 g/kg/day (> 4 hours/day).
♦ For fast refuelling and recovery, divide your food intake into five or six moderate-sized meals and snacks a day.
♦ Have a high carbohydrate meal 2–4 hours before exercise, followed by a snack containing 25–50 g of carbohydrate (for example one or two bananas) just before exercise.
♦ If you exercise hard for more than one hour, consuming an extra 30–60 g/hour carbohydrate in liquid or solid form will help to delay fatigue (500–1000 ml of isotonic sports drink or two/three bananas plus water).
♦ Have a high carbohydrate snack within two hours after exercise (for example a banana sandwich).
♦ Consume a variety of protein sources, including foods with a high biological value (milk, poultry, eggs) and foods with a low biological value (pulses, cereals).
♦ Keep your fat intake at below 30% of your energy intake, but do not reduce it too severely. Include the equivalent of 1–2 tablespoonfuls of vegetable oil, nuts or seeds a day in order to obtain the essential fatty acids and allow your body to absorb fat-soluble vitamins such as vitamin E.
♦ Aim to obtain all of your vitamins and minerals from nutrient-

rich foods. Consider a general multi-vitamin and mineral supplement if you are on a weight reducing diet, travel or eat out a lot. Antioxidant supplements may have health benefits and reduce the risk of free radical damage.
+ Do not take individual vitamin or mineral supplements indiscriminately without the advice of a sports nutritionist.

Further Reading

A. Bean, *The Complete Guide to Sports Nutrition* (A & C Black, 1993)
F. Brouns, *Nutritional Needs of Athletes* (Wiley, 1994)
Foods, Nutrition and Sports Performance (Journal of Sports Sciences Vol 9, 1991 – Special Issue)
International Journal of Sports Nutrition (Human Kinetics Publishers, inc.)
N. Clark, *Nancy Clark's Sports Nutrition Guidebook* (Leisure Press, Illinois, 1989)

2

NUTRITION DURING PREGNANCY

Anita Bean, BSc

It is generally accepted that a nutritious, balanced diet plays a vital role in both the development of a baby and in the mother's continued good health. There is also increasing evidence that dietary intake during pregnancy has long-term consequences for the child, affecting in particular the risk of heart disease, strokes, diabetes and bronchitis in later life (this concept is known as 'early programming').

Many exercising women worry that the physical and psychological demands of regular training may affect their chances of conception and of a successful pregnancy. They may ask themselves: 'Can a lower than average body weight and level of body fat have an adverse effect on the outcome of my pregnancy?' or 'Should I eat for two during this time, or try to restrict my weight gain to avoid unnecessary fat stores?'

This chapter will help to answer these and other questions by presenting the latest recommendations on pregnancy, nutrition and exercise and by offering practial advice on overcoming the dietary problems which are commonly encountered at this time. It will help you to understand and to meet your nutritional needs so that both you and your baby stand the best possible chance of good health both now and in the future.

Can I get pregnant if I have a low body fat level?

Low body fat and body weight are often associated with reduced sex hormone levels and reduced fertility. The threshold below which ovulation and menstruation stop (amenorrhoea) is usually between 15 and 20% fat or a BMI of less than 20. In order to become pregnant, a certain ratio of body fat to lean body mass is needed. Body fat is important for fertility because it is involved in the production of sex hormones which are responsible for ovulation. What's more, studies have shown that women with very low body fat tend to produce less potent forms of oestrogen.

If you have irregular or absent periods, gaining a little weight/ fat will increase your fertility and therefore your chances of successful conception. In practice, a reduction in training intensity and a small increase in food intake is sufficient to bring back normal menstrual cycles.

Your weight and body fat level before pregnancy are both important for your baby's development and pregnancy outcome. Studies have shown that a low pre-pregnancy weight increases the risk of babies with a low birth weight.

So make sure that your weight and body fat are within a healthy range before you plan to get pregnant, as this will help to bring about conception and to increase the likelihood of having a baby of optimal weight.

Table 1: *Body composition changes*

Body component	Increase in weight
Baby	3.4 kg
Placenta	0.65 kg
Amniotic fluid	0.8 kg
Uterus	0.97 kg
Breast	0.41 kg
Blood	1.25 kg
Extracellular fluid	1.68 kg
Fat	3.35 kg
Total	**12.5 kg**

How much weight should I put on?

On average, most women gain around 12.5 kg (28 lb) during a full-term pregnancy of 40 weeks, although anywhere between 11.5 and 16 kg (25–35 lb) is considered healthy. About one quarter of this (3–4 kg/6–9 lb) will be the weight of your baby; about half (6 kg/13 lb) will be pregnancy-related tissues (placenta, amniotic fluid, uterus, breast tissue and extra blood); and about one quarter (3–4 kg/6–9 lb) will be laid down as a fat store.

This fat is deposited mainly subcutaneously in the upper thighs, hips and abdomen under the influence of the hormone *progesterone*. Most fat deposition occurs in mid pregnancy. The idea is that it acts as a buffer of energy stores for late pregnancy and breast feeding when the energy demands of the baby are highest.

Interestingly, fat mobilisation starts in the latter stages of pregnancy and continues for a short while after the birth, as levels of the hormone lactogen rise. In other words, various pregnancy hormones encourage your body to lay down fat mid-term and then mobilise it late and post-term.

The amount of fat stored varies enormously. In practice, some women gain far more than 3–4 kg – up to 20 kg in extreme cases! In 1990 the Institute of Medicine of the US National Academy of Sciences issued guidelines for optimum weight gain. They suggested that what you should gain depends on how heavy you are at the start of your pregnancy. If you are overweight, you should aim to gain a little less than the normal recommendation. If you are underweight, than you should aim to 'catch up' by gaining more than 28 lb. This greatly improves your chances of having an easy pregnancy.

Table 2: *Guidelines for weight gain during pregnancy*
(US National Academy of Sciences, 1990)

Underweight (BMI < 19.8)	28–40 lb	12.5–18 kg
Normal weight (BMI 19.8–26)	25–35 lb	11.5–16 kg
Overweight (BMI 26–29)	15–25 lb	7–11.5 kg
Obese (BMI > 30)	13 lb (min.)	6 kg (min.)
$$BMI = \dfrac{\text{weight (kg)}}{\text{height (m)}^2}$$		

What are the dangers of putting on too much weight?

Obviously, it is important to avoid putting on too much fat. Being overweight and gaining too much weight in pregnancy increases the risk of *gestational diabetes* (a mild form of diabetes). This is usually only temporary but may occasionally turn out to be more of a serious long-term problem. There is also the danger of developing high blood pressure or *pre-eclampsia*, which is associated with premature delivery. Very overweight women are more likely to have extra-large babies which may need forceps or caesarean delivery. So, follow the guidelines given in table 2 at the bottom of the previous page.

What dangers are associated with being underweight in pregnancy?

Being underweight (BMI < 20) or restricting your weight gain if you are not overweight will affect your developing baby. Studies have shown that a low pregnancy weight-gain may seriously retard your baby's growth in the womb and that this can have adverse consequences on later growth (possibly also on neuro-behavioural development). The baby is more likely to be underweight when born and shorter in length than normal. Head circumference is also likely to be smaller.

The important message is: if you are underweight, make sure you put on a minimum of 28 lb. If you are normal weight, do not overly restrict your weight gain: aim for around 28 lb. If you are overweight, you should aim for a slightly smaller weight gain but speak to your doctor or dietitian first.

How many calories should you eat?

During early pregnancy, the extra amount of food energy required is very small indeed. So, contrary to popular belief, you don't need to eat extra calories at this time. Only during the last three months is there a substantial increase in energy needs as the baby grows larger and additional pregnancy-related tissues are laid down. The Department of Health recommends an extra 200 calories a day at this time. Again, this is not a hard and fast rule as it depends on your weight at the start of pregnancy. Over-weight women may need fewer than this; underweight women may need more.

Will my metabolism change?

It is a common misconception that your metabolic rate drops when you are pregnant. Many women attribute their excess weight (fat) gain to a reduction in their metabolic rate, but this has been shown to be completely untrue.

Researchers at the Dunn Clinical Nutrition Centre monitored the metabolic rates of British and Gambian women before and during their pregnancy. Interestingly, they found that the meta-bolic rate of British women who were slightly plump actually *increased* whilst they were pregnant! The metabolism of very thin British and Gambian women slowed during pregnancy, presumably due to a need for energy conservation. In other words, the body is remarkably adaptive to a wide range of calorie intakes.

Carbohydrate, fat and protein metabolism changes during pregnancy due to alterations in hormone levels. Your body's main priority is to help ensure a steady supply of glucose for the baby, so your body adapts to make better use of fats for fuel. Hormonal changes also make sure that your lean tissue is conserved and not broken down for energy unless it proves absolutely necessary.

Doesn't pregnancy give you a weight problem for life?

It is quite normal and necessary to gain some extra fat during pregnancy. This is in preparation for breastfeeding and is also nature's safety precaution in case of famine during later preg-nancy. Fat gain should amount to 3–4 kg, on average, and most (if not all) will be quickly utilised for milk production when you start breastfeeding.

However, there is no reason why pregnancy should give you a long-term weight problem. It has been shown that women who gained a lot of excess weight during pregnancy were already overweight or had in any case been battling with a weight problem before they became pregnant. Another theory is that before they marry or become pregnant many women suppress their weight by dieting to please the opposite sex. Once they are pregnant and see their body expanding, they give up the dieting battle and use pregnancy as the perfect excuse to over-indulge. Hence, the excess weight gain.

Any excess fat gained during pregnancy over and above the normal 3–4 kg can be safely and gradually lost through a combination of a healthy low fat diet and regular exercise, once breast-feeding has ceased (*see* chapter 7). It is not recommended to restrict calorie intake during breastfeeding because you risk not obtaining sufficient amounts of key nutrients (e.g. calcium, essential fatty acids) needed for breast milk production.

Is it dangerous to restrict my food intake during pregnancy?

Restricting your food intake can lead to all sorts of problems unless you take proper professional advice from a nutritionist. It is often difficult for lean athletes to accept increases in their body weight and fat. You may feel tempted to restrict your fat gain by restricting your food intake, but you may encounter a number of potentially serious problems.

First, you can affect the growth and development of your baby. In general, the lower your calorie intake, the lower the weight of your baby. For example, in one study carried out on women living in Hackney, London, low-birth-weight babies were more common in those women who had the lowest daily calorie intake (1600 kcal).

Second, if you skip a meal or leave a long gap between meals your blood sugar levels will fall. This can have harmful consequences on your developing baby, who relies on a steady supply of blood sugar from your shared bloodstream. Remember, your baby has no energy stores and is therefore totally reliant on a constant supply of fuel and nutrients from you.

Third, there is a danger that you may not get enough nutrients to sustain your body's stores *and* to feed your baby. Generally, your baby will take what he or she needs from your body, but if your stores run out then he or she may suffer too. The end result could be depleted iron stores for you and a greater danger of early osteoporosis unless you keep up your intake of key nutrients such as iron and calcium.

Do I need extra fat?

Certain types of fats are especially important in pregnancy, so you will have to make sure that you include these regularly in your diet. The two essential fatty acids (linoleic acid and linolenic acid) cannot be made in the body. They are converted to arachidonic acid and docosahexanoic acid respectively which are essential for brain and central nervous system development. They are also needed for cell development and healthy sperm (make sure your partner includes them in his diet!). A deficiency of these fatty acids may therefore affect your baby's brain development.

Athletes who follow a very low fat diet *must* ensure that they include essential fatty acids in their diet and this is particularly vital prior to conception and during pregnancy. This may mean slightly increasing the amount of fat you normally eat. Good sources of essential fatty acids include vegetable oils (sunflower, rapeseed), oily fish (sardines, mackerel), nuts and seeds. The equivalent of a tablespoon of oil or 25 g (1 oz) of nuts or seeds a day will give you enough essential fatty acids. Experts also recommend oily fish at least once a week.

Do I need extra vitamins?

During pregnancy there is an increased need for most vitamins and minerals, especially during the last three months. Most of the baby's needs are met by your existing stores of minerals and fat-soluble vitamins; nevertheless, the Department of Health advises a modest increase in your intake of thiamin, riboflavin, folate, and vitamins A, D and C.

In theory, you should be able to get all you need from your diet, but multivitamin and mineral supplements may be a sensible precaution. Vitamin supplements are available to all pregnant women free or at a reduced cost from ante-natal clinics. Ask your doctor or dietitian for advice.

Should I take folic acid supplements?

The Department of Health advises any woman planning a pregnancy to take a supplement of 400 µg (0.4 mg) of folic acid a day. This is because a deficiency has been linked with a greater risk of neutral tube defects such as spina bifida in newborn babies. Studies have shown that high intakes of this B vitamin (from supplements) taken prior to conception and during early pregnancy can reduce the risks. Although women who have already had an affected baby are at greater risk, the Department of Health recommendation applies to all women because 95% of pregnancies affected by a NTD are a first occurence.

The average adult's intake of folic acid is only about 130 µg a day. You can increase your intake by eating more folic acid-rich foods, eating foods fortified with folic acid (some breakfast cereals and bread) or taking folic acid supplements. Fruit, vegetables and yeast extract are the best food sources and offer a range of other nutrients too. Refer to table 3 for more information.

Table 3: *The folic acid content of various foods*

Food	Portion size	Folic acid (µg/portion)
Broccoli	100 g	64
Baked potato	200 g	88
Beetroot	100 g	110
Brussels sprouts	100 g	110
Cabbage	100 g	29
Mushrooms (raw)	50 g	22
Spinach	100 g	90
Banana	One	15
Oranges	One	50
Bran Flakes (fortified)	40 g	100
Cornflakes (fortified)	40 g	100
Yeast extract	4 g	40
Chick peas (boiled)	150 g	81

Do I need extra minerals?

There are no official recommendations for extra minerals during pregnancy, but it is definitely a good idea to make sure you get a little extra from your diet to safeguard your stores.

Calcium

Calcium is needed for bone and teeth development and there is evidence that it may also be important in regulating blood pressure during pregnancy. Calcium requirements increase during pregnancy, particularly in the last 10 weeks when the baby's bones are growing fast. However, there is no recommendation to increase your dietary intake as your baby's increased needs are met from your existing calcium stores (bones) and also by increasing calcium absorption from food.

Iron

Iron is needed for the manufacture of haemoglobin in red blood cells. More red blood cells are made during pregnancy to help carry oxygen to the baby. About one third of your iron stores are used for this purpose, so it is important that you get enough iron in your diet to prevent anaemia. The absorption of iron from food increases naturally during pregnancy from about 7–10% up to 30–40% towards the end in order to meet your increased needs.

The RNI is 14.8 mg, and there is no official recommendation for an increased dietary intake, nor for routine supplements. However, many exercisers tend to have low iron stores (although they are not anaemic) which may put them at risk of iron-deficiency anaemia during or after pregnancy. Iron supplements may therefore be advisable so you should check with your doctor. Refer to table 4 for more information.

Zinc

Zinc is involved in cell division and so is essential for your baby's growth. As with iron, this additional zinc comes from your body's stores and through increased intestinal absorption. So there is no official dietary recommendation for increased intake or supple-

Table 4: *The iron content of various foods*

Food	Portion size	Iron (mg/portion)
Beef (average cut)	100 g	2.8
Chicken (meat only)	150 g	1.2
Sardines	50 g	2.3
Lentils (cooked)	120 g	4.0
Baked beans	200 g	2.8
Eggs	2	1.6
Weetabix	2	3.0
Broccoli	100 g	1.0
Spinach	100 g	1.7
Wholemeal bread	2 slices	1.3

ments. Zinc is also needed for health sperm, so make sure your partner has a plentiful supply if you are planning a pregnancy!

However, if you have been advised to take iron supplements, you may need to take zinc supplements too or a multi-vitamin supplement since a high iron intake can reduce zinc absorption. Consult a sports nutritionist if in doubt.

What about food cravings?

Changes in taste and appetite are common during pregnancy, though whether there is a true physiological basis to this remains open to debate. Many women develop an increased appetite and experience a ravenous desire (craving) for certain foods. If your diet is otherwise well balanced then this is unlikely to be a problem, especially if your craving is for a fairly healthy food. If you must give in to less healthy cravings, do so only in moderation and make sure that you are still getting enough nutrients from other foods. A good idea is to try healthier options of less nourishing cravings, e.g. scone instead of cake.

Many women find they go off certain fatty and fried foods, alcohol, meat, coffee or spicy foods in the first few months.

Table 5: *Food sources of special nutrients (vitamins and minerals)*

Calcium	Low fat milk, yoghurt, cheese, fromage frais, dark green vegetables, beans, lentils, almonds, sardines, prawns, figs
Iron	Red meat, liver, wholemeal bread, wholegrain or fortified breakfast cereals, dark green vegetables, beans, lentils
Zinc	Red meat, wholegrain bread and cereals, nuts, seeds, eggs
Folic acid	Green leafy vegetables, liver, wholegrain cereals, eggs, beans, lentils, bananas
Vitamin D	Oily fish, eggs, margarine, fortified breakfast cereals
B vitamins	Wholegrain cereals, pulses, nuts, meat, milk, cheese
Vitamin C	Strawberries, raspberries, black-currants, oranges, green vegetables, peppers, orange juice, tomatoes

Again, this is not a problem provided that the rest of your diet is nutritious and you drink plenty of other fluids such as herb/fruit teas, water and diluted fruit juice instead of coffee and tea.

What about morning sickness?

More than half of all pregnant women suffer from morning sickness, nausea or heartburn. These symptoms are thought to be due to dramatic increases in certain hormones, such as human chorionic growth hormone (HCG) produced by the placenta.

Don't worry about your baby, who will draw on your nutrient stores and be well protected against deficiencies. Try to eat small, high carbohydrate snacks at regular intervals to ease nausea: a roll with banana, breakfast cereal, dried fruit, yoghurt, or rice cakes

Table 6: *Sample Daily Eating Plan for a Pregnant Woman*

(Suitable for vegetarians and meat-eaters)	
Breakfast:	50 g (2 oz) Bran Flakes, one chopped banana and 300 ml low-fat milk *or* two to three slices of wholemeal toast, marmite and fruit
Snack:	One piece of fruit; one yoghurt or low fat milk drink
Lunch:	Large jacket potato with 100 g (4 oz) of tuna *or* baked beans on wholemeal toast Side salad with 1 tbsp oil/vinegar dressing Fromage frais and fresh fruit
Snack:	Bagel or fruit scone Diluted fruit juice
Dinner:	200 g (8 oz) of cooked pasta with tomato and lean mince/fish/ham sauce *or* pasta with lentil/vegetable sauce Large portion of vegetables or salad Rice pudding with fruit
Energy: 2200 kcal; carbohydrate: 60%; protein: 20%; fat: 20%	

with fruit spread. To reduce morning sickness, try crystallised ginger, ginger biscuits, plain biscuits or toast. And if you fancy strange food combinations, e.g. marmite and gherkin sandwiches, go ahead. It's better to eat something than nothing at all. Milk-based drinks can alleviate heartburn. Make your own milkshake from low fat milk, fruit and yoghurt, or use a commercial mix and add milk. Drink plenty of fluids too.

Should I avoid caffeine?

There is no convincing evidence that caffeine in moderation has any adverse effect on pregnancy. Some early studies suggested that high intakes reduced fertility and birth weight and increased the risk of birth defects. However, these have not been proved and more recent, more comprehensive studies have found no ill-effects at all.

During pregnancy your body metabolises caffeine more slowly, especially during the last three months. Caffeine can pass freely across the placenta but there is no evidence of any harm caused by moderate intakes. Many pregnant women find that they develop an aversion to coffee and tea in any case, but the physiological reason for this is not known.

So, if you like drinking coffee and tea, there is no reason why you should not continue to take in moderate amounts – the equivalent of 4–5 cups a day will not do any harm.

Can I drink alcohol?

The occasional drink certainly won't harm you or your baby, but heavy drinking (more than 30 units a week) can lead to stunted growth and retarded mental development – a condition sometimes called *Foetal Alcohol Syndrome*. Alcohol can pass from your bloodstream across the placenta into your baby's blood, so high levels can affect his or her development.

According to the Royal College of Physicians, it is safest to avoid alcohol altogether, especially during the first three months. After that, limit yourself to one or two units a day once or twice a week. One unit is equivalent to half a pint of beer, one glass of wine or one 'pub measure' of spirits.

Is vitamin A harmful in pregnancy?

Vitamin A itself is not harmful; indeed it is essential for a healthy pregnancy as it is needed for proper cell division and development. The reason why it has hit the headlines recently is because of a few cases reported in the US where mega-dose supplements of vitamin A (more than 8000–10,000 μg per day) have led to birth abnormalities. However, these doses were more than ten times the daily requirement (700 μg/day).

As a safety precaution the Department of Health advises pregnant women to avoid vitamin A supplements and fish liver oil capsules (unless advised by a doctor). They also recommend avoiding liver (and products made from it such as liver pâté and liver sausage) because they can sometimes contain very high concentrations of vitamin A.

There is no risk from other vitamin A sources such as milk, cheese, eggs and carrots because they contain much smaller concentrations. Only one case of vitamin A toxicity has been recorded in a pregnant woman who ate too much liver. So, in reality, the risk of overdosing on vitamin A is very small indeed!

Am I or my baby at risk from listeriosis?

Listeriosis is an illness caused by the listeria bacteria which contaminate certain foods. It is quite rare and produces flu-like symptoms. It is of concern to pregnant women because it can cause miscarriage, still-birth or severe illness in the new-born baby.

Unlike most other bacteria, listeria can multiply at the low temperatures found in refrigerators. It can be a problem with certain cheeses contaminated after manufacture, because they are kept for fairly long periods at low temperatures thus giving the bacteria a chance to multiply. The Department of Health advises that pregnant women:

◆ avoid mould-ripened soft cheeses such as camembert and brie, and also blue-veined cheeses such as blue Stilton (hard cheeses, cottage cheese and processed cheese are fine);
◆ re-heat 'cooked-chilled' foods (for example ready-made meals) and ready-to-eat poultry until they are piping hot;
◆ avoid pâté and under-cooked poultry or meat products;
◆ wash salads, vegetables and fruit thoroughly;
◆ check the 'Use By' dates of chilled food;
◆ store cooked and raw foods separately in the fridge.

Am I at risk from salmonella poisoning?

Pregnant women are more prone to salmonella poisoning. This won't harm your baby, but it can cause sickness and diarrhoea in you. Reduce the risks by:

- avoiding raw or lightly cooked eggs and products made with them (for example mayonnaise, mousse, home-made, uncooked cheesecake);
- make sure eggs are cooked until both the white and yolk are solid;
- avoid undercooked chicken;
- avoid cross-contamination of uncooked chicken and other foods – keep work surfaces clean and store raw and cooked foods separately in the fridge;
- reheat cooked chicken until it is piping hot.

Should I stop exercising when I'm pregnant?

There is no reason to stop exercising during pregnancy if you are accustomed to regular training. You can certainly continue to train provided you feel well and are not excessively tired or nauseous, although you may have to make a few modifications to your usual programme. Indeed, exercise during pregnancy brings many physiological and psychological benefits. It is not advisable, however, for very unfit women or those who have not exercised regularly previously to embark on an intensive programme.

The important difference is that you should now aim to *maintain* rather than *improve* your fitness. In practice, this means reducing your training intensity and volume to a level lower than before. This will not result in a decrease in fitness because your body is naturally undergoing a training effect during pregnancy. Large increases in oestrogen output encourage the development of bone strength and lean tissue mass, including skeletal muscle. The heart muscle becomes stronger, increasing stroke and blood volume. Raised levels of progesterone relax the smooth muscles, including those surrounding the blood vessels, allowing them to accommodate this increased blood volume. All of these changes mimic those resulting from regular physical training!

As pregnancy progresses, gradually reduce your training intensity and volume. Many conditioned women find they can continue exercising until the thirtieth week or longer. There is no recommended cut-off date before the birth but you should listen carefully to your body, observe the precautions detailed in this chapter and stop exercising if you notice any of the symptoms listed in table 7 or if the first stage of labour commences.

What are the benefits of regular exercise during pregnancy?

Regular exercise will maintain good stamina, boosting your ability to deal with the physical demands of pregnancy. Your posture will improve, reducing posture-related problems such as backache, joint problems and lordosis (excessive arching of the lower back). Common pregnancy ailments such as tiredness, nausea, constipation, varicose veins, cramps and water retention will be alleviated, and the likelihood of excessive fat gain lessened. You will also be paving the way for an easier labour.

Regular exercise brings many psychological benefits, such as reduced stress and anxiety, enhanced feelings of wellbeing, improved self-esteem and body image.

There is evidence that exercise in early pregnancy stimulates placental growth and that continued exercise throughout the term may improve placental function by about 30%, thereby enhancing placental blood flow to the developing foetus.

Are there any special precautions I should take when exercising?

You should avoid any activity that places excessive pressure or stress upon your joints. Avoid overextending any joint or any activity that causes excessive movement around your joints, as the ligaments (which support the joints) become softer and more lax owing to the effects of the hormone *relaxin*. The joints most at risk are the pelvic joints and the sacro-ileac (lower back) joint, particularly in the second and third trimesters of pregnancy.

For this reason, it is best to avoid prolonged high impact activities such as running (and any sports which include running), jumping, plyometrics and high impact aerobics. You should also avoid using very heavy weights when weight training and pay extra attention to correct technique. To minimise the stress on your joints, it is advisable to modify your programme to include low impact activities such as swimming, walking, low impact aerobics, light to moderate weight training, light circuit training, aqua-aerobics and any sport that doesn't involve much running or jumping.

Avoid repetitive stress to your joints and muscles by varying the muscle groups used within a single training session (e.g. by combining lower body and upper body exercises) and also by varying the types of activities in your programme, i.e. cross training.

Good technique is even more important during pregnancy to ensure good joint alignment (e.g. hips, knees, ankles), and avoid unbalanced loads (e.g. during resistance training).

It is important both for your body and your developing baby to ensure your core body temperature does not exceed 38°C. Overheating, or hyperthermia, may, in theory, harm the development of your baby and result in foetal growth retardation. To avoid thermal stress, the American College of Obstetricians and Gynaecologists recommends that you should limit the duration of strenuous activity to 15 minutes and make sure your heart rate does not exceed 140 beats per minute for an extended period of time. Other sensible precautions include exercising at a low or submaximal level (less than 65% of VO_2 max), ensuring your surroundings are well ventilated and not too warm, keeping well hydrated by drinking plenty of fluids, and allowing sufficient cool-down time after training. The risk of thermal stress is smaller for well-conditioned women as they are better able to thermoregulate than those new to exercise.

Think consciously about reducing your training intensity. During pregnancy it is easy to underestimate your exertion due to increased levels of beta-endorphins ('pain-killer' hormones produced by the brain), which decrease your perceived rate of exertion.

Should I avoid any particular exercises?

The American College of Obstetricians and Gynaecologists recommends avoiding any exercises performed in the supine (lying down) position after the fourth month of pregnancy. This is because of the increased weight of the uterus pressing down on the *vena cava* (the main vein that returns blood to the heart) which can cause a drop in blood pressure, dizziness and faintness.

For most women, after about the twentieth week of pregnancy the abdominus recti separates longitudinally to accommodate the size of the baby. Once this has occurred, you should avoid intensive abdominal exercises as these cause uneven pressure on the recti, resulting in a 'dome' along the *linea alba* (central connective tissue). Curl-ups should therefore be avoided once the abdomen can no longer be kept flat in the supine position. A recommended alternative abdominal exercise is trunk curls, which are performed on all fours.

Avoid any hyperextension (arching) of the back as this will over-stretch the softened ligaments of the sacro-ileac joint, resulting in back pain and lordosis. The American College of Obstetricians and Gynaecologists also advises against increased intra-abdominal pressure or straining (e.g. when lifting heavy weights or performing resistance exercises) as this can raise blood pressure and restrict blood supply to the foetus. Avoid isometric (static or held) exercises, e.g. holding arms overhead for a long period, as these can also increase blood pressure.

What about the pelvic floor muscles?

The pelvic floor muscles hang like a taut hammock between the pubic bone at the front and the coccyx at the back. These support the abdominal contents (i.e. uterus, bladder, intestines, etc.). During pregnancy and labour they come under extra stress, so it is important to help strengthen them by including pelvic floor exercises (Kegal exercises) in your daily routine. This will help prevent some of the common discomforts such as haemorrhoids, constipation and urinary incontinence, and also prepare the way for an easier childbirth.

Is there any other advice to follow?

Wear a good supportive bra and correct footwear during exercise to help avoid back and joint problems.

Pay special attention to your posture at all times as this will help minimise strain on your lower back caused by the weight of your uterus pulling down. When standing, lengthen the spine, keep the abdominals taut, your shoulders down and chest lifted. Your knees should be relaxed. When sitting, keep your spine upright and supported in the region of your lower back, and the back of your thighs in contact with the seat. Do not slouch forward.

Table 7: *Reasons to stop exercising*

If you experience any of the following symptoms, stop exercising and consult your doctor or midwife:

- ♦ vaginal bleeding
- ♦ very rapid heart beat
- ♦ dizziness or faintness
- ♦ pelvic pain
- ♦ nausea
- ♦ shortness of breath
- ♦ uterine contractions
- ♦ back pain
- ♦ abdominal pain
- ♦ excessive fatigue

Learn to listen to your body. Do not exercise if you feel unduly tired, nauseous or faint. Do not push yourself too hard, and stop if you feel uncomfortable, notice any spotting or experience any pain, particularly in the pelvic region.

SUMMARY

- ♦ Low body fat and weight are usually associated with reduced sex hormone levels and reduced fertility. Chances of conception decrease below a threshold of 15–20% fat or a BMI of 20.
- ♦ A low pre-pregnancy weight may increase the risk of having a low-birth-weight baby.
- ♦ The average weight gain is 11.5–16 kg: underweight women should aim to gain slightly more; overweight women should aim to gain slightly less.
- ♦ Being underweight (BMI < 20) or intentionally restricting your weight gain in pregnancy can restrict the growth and development of your baby and have adverse long-term consequences.

- Extra calories are not required until the last three months of pregnancy, when an additional 200 calories per day are recommended.
- Weight problems post-pregnancy are not inevitable: there is no evidence that pregnancy causes a decreased metabolic rate or excessive fat deposition.
- Your diet should contain enough essential fatty acids to support the growth and development of your baby's brain and central nervous system.
- There is an increased need for most vitamins and minerals, but most of these are met by the baby drawing on your exisiting stores and through increased intestinal absorption. The most important ones include calcium, iron, zinc, folic acid, vitamin C, vitamin D and the B vitamins.
- You may continue a regular training programme throughout pregnancy, provided you feel well, gradually reducing the training intensity and volume as pregnancy progresses.
- Aim to maintain rather than increase your fitness.
- Avoid any activity that places excessive pressure, stress or movement on any joint because the ligaments are more lax during pregnancy. Avoid repetitive stress to your joints and pay extra attention to correct technique.
- Avoid thermal stress by using low or sub-maximal intensity activities, limiting strenuous activity to 15 minutes duration and ensuring your heart rate does not often exceed 140 bpm.
- It is recommended that pregnant women avoid any supine exercises, particularly abdominal exercises performed in the supine position, after the twentieth week.

PRACTICAL POINTS

- If you are planning to become pregnant and have irregular or absent periods, you may have to reduce your training intensity and/or increase your body fat a little. This will improve your chances of conception and help ensure an optimal birth weight for your baby.
- Include plenty of folate-rich foods (fruit and vegetables) in your

diet and take a supplement containing 400 µg of folic acid until the twelfth week of pregnancy.

♦ Do not attempt to restrict your food intake or go on a diet during pregnancy. This may mean your baby will be born shorter and lighter than normal.

♦ Include the equivalent of one tablespoon of oil or 25 g of nuts or seeds in your daily diet, and oily fish at least once a week.

♦ Eat plenty of vitamin and mineral-rich foods. Each day, include at least five portions of fruit and vegetables; 5–11 portions of cereals/starchy vegetables; three portions of low fat dairy products; and two portions of protein-rich foods (for example meat, poultry and pulses).

♦ Ideally, avoid alcohol for the first three months. After that the occasional drink is fine.

♦ Avoid vitamin A supplements, liver and liver products.

♦ Concentrate on low impact activities such as swimming, walking, low impact aerobics, moderate-light weight training, light circuit training, and avoid prolonged high impact activities (e.g. running, jumping). Vary the activities in your routine.

♦ Listen to your body and do not exercise if you feel fatigued, nauseous or dizzy. Do not exercise to the point of exhaustion.

♦ Reduce the risk of thermal stress by ensuring your body temperature does not exceed 38°C. Drink plenty of fluids before, during and after exercise, monitor your heart beat, exercise in well-ventilated surroundings and allow extra time for cooling down.

♦ Make sure you avoid any hyperextention of the lower back and pay strict attention to posture at all times.

Further reading

National Dairy Council, *Maternal and Fetal Nutrition* (Fact File No. 11, 1994)

British Nutrition Foundation, *Nutrition in Pregnancy* (Briefing Paper, 1994)

IRON AND SPORTS ANAEMIA

Dr Eric Watts

Dr Eric J. Watts DM FRCP MRCPath Dip Hlth Mgt is Consultant Haematologist at Basildon Hospital and his research experience includes the effects of exercise on the blood. He is a keen runner and contributes to various sports medicine courses and conferences.

This chapter will describe the role of iron in the body, iron balance in female exercisers and the effects of sports competition on iron status. It will also review the evidence for or against iron *supplementation*, i.e. taking additional iron.

Why do we need iron?

Iron *is* essential for life. It combines with oxygen, carrying it around the body and into the cells where energy is released by oxygenating (or *burning*) the carbon and hydrogen derived from food. Most iron in the blood is in the form of *haemoglobin*, the material which colours the cells red (*see* fig. 1). The equivalent compound in the muscles is *myoglobin*.

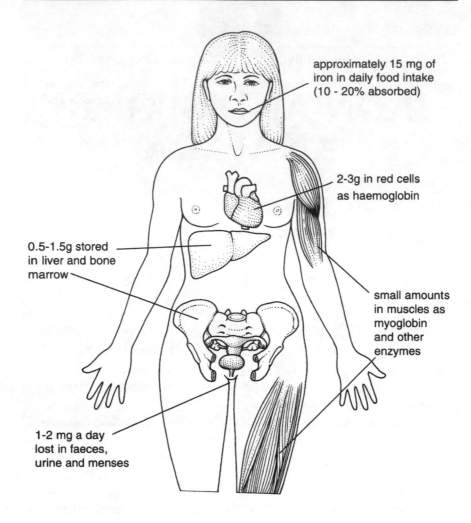

approximately 15 mg of
iron in daily food intake
(10 - 20% absorbed)

2-3g in red cells
as haemoglobin

0.5-1.5g stored
in liver and bone
marrow

small amounts
in muscles as
myoglobin
and other
enzymes

1-2 mg a day
lost in faeces,
urine and menses

Figure 1: *Iron deposits in the body*

Although essential for life, iron is also potentially toxic if it is
present in certain tissues in excess, especially the heart, liver and
pancreas. Excess iron in the body causes the rare disease of
haemochromatosis which causes patients to develop liver damage,
diabetes and heart failure. The body does not have an effective
way of getting rid of excess iron, so it prevents overload by
regulating the amount absorbed from the gut, which is normally
around 10%. With the average western diet, this is sufficient to
supply 1 mg of iron per day which meets the needs of most men,

Table 1: Factors influencing iron absorption

Absorption is increased by:	Absorption is decreased by:
♦ Ferrous (*haeme*) iron, e.g. in meat, fish, poultry and organ meat	♦ Ferric (*non-haeme*) iron, e.g. in vegetables, pulses, cereals and nuts
♦ Acidic environment as in stomach	♦ Alkaline environment as in duodenum
♦ Vitamin C	♦ Tannin, e.g. tea
♦ Some sugars, e.g. fructose, sorbitol	♦ Phosphates, e.g. egg yolk
♦ Iron deficiency state	♦ Other substances such as phytate, bran and inorganic elements such as calcium
♦ Pregnancy	♦ Iron overload
♦ Fasting/dieting	♦ Illness due to infection or inflammation, e.g. arthritis

and non-menstruating and non-pregnant females. Normally, iron is lost from the body in cells which are shed from the skin and from the gastroentestrinal tract, i.e. from the stomach and bowels. Menstruation increases the requirement for iron to the equivalent of 2–3 mg of iron per day. Women with heavy periods will require more. During pregnancy the requirement for iron is also 2 mg a day (*see* table 1).

In addition to menstrual blood loss, blood may be lost through medical conditions such as ulcers or piles. When blood is lost from piles it is always obvious, but blood can be lost from a duodenal ulcer, which may not cause symptoms, and the blood – being mixed with the other bowel contents – might not be apparent. Hence anaemia may often occur without any obvious cause.

What is anaemia?

Anaemia literally means lack of blood. It is normally defined as *that situation in which the haemoglobin concentration is insufficient to meet the body's needs*. (The normal level of haemoglobin for women is 11.5–16.5 g/dl.) Anaemia may also be characterised by a low level of *ferritin*, which is the storage form of iron. This indicates that iron stores are being depleted. (The normal level of ferritin in the blood is greater than 15 µg/litre.)

The characteristic symptoms of anaemia are fatigue and breathlessness during exercise. Unfortunately these symptoms are not specific to anaemia. Tiredness and fatigue, for example, are very common symptoms in healthy people and can result from stress as well as from physical illness. Anaemia may cause poor athletic performance and is worth considering when there has been an unexplained loss of form or training/competition has been impaired for some inexplicable reason.

Table 2: *Dietary sources of iron*

Iron is well absorbed from: (*high bioavailability*)	Iron is less well absorbed from: (*moderate-low bioavailability*)
Meat (especially red meat) Poultry Fish Liver and other organ meat	Cereals (breakfast cereals, oatmeal, bread, rice, pasta) Beans (including baked beans) Peas Lentils Nuts Dried fruits (apricots, raisins, dates, prunes, sultanas) Fortified TVP mince and tofu Dark green leafy vegetables Egg yolks Treacle (Licquorice Allsorts)

Practical tip: try to include iron-rich foods (which are readily absorbed) in your diet **every day**. If you are a vegetarian and do not consume foods with a high bioavailability (i.e. meat, fish, offal, etc.), then ensure that you do include plenty of non-meat iron sources. Because the iron in these foods tends to be less readily absorbed, it is important to avoid any practices which further hinder absorption - *see* table 1 for further reference. Try also to combine non-meat sources of iron with vitamin C, since this will improve iron absorption.

Which foods contain iron?

Foods rich in iron include meat – particularly red meat – poultry and fish. Although vegetables are not as rich in iron as meat, good vegetable sources are peas and beans (*see* also table 2).

A number of factors affect the absorption of iron. The chemical state of the iron is important: it is absorbed more efficiently if it exists in a reduced (or ferrous) form as it is in meat, poultry, fish and liver. This is sometimes called *haeme* iron. If it is in the oxidised (or ferric) form, as is found in vegetables, it is absorbed less readily and is known as *non-haeme* iron. It is also absorbed better in an acidic environment, for example if it is taken with lemon or orange juice which contains absorbic acid (vitamin C). Certain foods contain substances which form complexes with iron and reduce absorption, for example tea (tannin), chapatis (phytates) and rhubarb (oxalic acid). Meat encourages the absorption of iron by stimulating the stomach to produce acid (*see* table 1).

The recommended intake of iron (Reference Nutrient Intake or RNI) for females is 14.8 mg, but many women do not eat this much. The body can increase the proportion of iron absorbed when iron deficiency occurs by up to a maximum of 37%; this explains why some women who eat less than the RNI are not iron deficient. Iron deficiency is nevertheless very common: researchers from the University of Southampton report that one third of normal women have no iron stores.

Table 3 lists the amount of iron in common foods. Use this to calculate your daily iron intake.

How does sport and exercise affect iron systems?

For the majority of people, sport and exercise have no effect on their iron status, but there are some exceptions. All athletes who undertake endurance training to the extent that they develop 'cardiac conditioning', i.e. a fall in their resting pulse rate, will develop an increase in their blood volume, which can result in a syndrome called *sports anaemia*, in which the haemoglobin concentration falls from the average of 14 to 13.5g/dl. This syndrome is well recognised and there have been many suggestions as to the cause. Some of the suggestions have led to unnecessary anxiety and concern amongst exercisers, coaches and instructors, often

Table 3: *The iron content of various foods*

Food	Iron (mg per portion)	Portion/size
Liver (chicken)	4.75	per 50 g slice
Minced beef (cooked)	3.10	per 100 g portion
Sirloin steak (cooked)	3.80	per large portion (200 g)
Chicken (roast)	0.8	per four slices
Cod (baked)	0.4	per fillet (100 g)
Mackerel (smoked)	1.20	per small fillet (100 g)
Bran Flakes	6.0	per small bowl (30 g)
Cornflakes	2.0	per small bowl (30 g)
Baked beans	2.8	per half medium tin (200 g)
Red kidney beans	4.0	per half medium tin (200 g)
Brown bread	1.3	per two average slices
White bread	1.0	per two average slices
Brown rice (raw)	0.7	per 2 oz portion (uncooked)
White rice (raw)	0.25	per 2 oz portion (uncooked)
Raisins	1.9	per two tablespoons (50 g)
Prunes	2.6	per 10 prunes (100 g)
Dry roasted peanuts	0.5	per small packet (25 g)
Cashew nuts (roasted)	1.6	per small packet (25 g)
Broccoli (boiled)	1.0	per normal portion (40 g)
Cabbage (boiled)	0.3	per two large tablespoons (40 g)

The Reference Nutrient Intake (RNI) for the female population is **14.8 mg per day**. Use this table to assess your iron intake
Note: the iron content of different cuts of meat and varying forms of other foods may differ, so use this table only as a rough guide

leading to unnecessary treatments. It seems paradoxical that when most other physiological measurements show improved function after training, the haemoglobin level should fall, but studies on runners, rowers, cyclists, swimmers and walkers have consistently shown this to be the case.

What causes sports anaemia?

Iron deficiency is often considered to be the cause of sports anaemia and blood loss may occasionally occur in runners. Blood in the urine (*haematuria*) is particularly easy to detect. It has been reported many times in runners covering distances greater than 10 km. Investigations with a cystoscope, an instrument which allows the bladder to be inspected from the inside, have shown bruising of the lining of the bladder, presumably as a result of the upper wall of the bladder being repeatedly pressed against the lower wall by the abdominal contents bouncing up and down with each footstrike. Normally the haematuria ceases within hours of completion of a run and the amount of blood loss is seldom significant. One expert has suggested that runners should prevent this from occurring by running with a full bladder – needless to say, few runners have taken this advice!

Haemoglobinuria is another well recognised complication of running or marching. This condition is different from haematuria in that haematuria causes the urine to take on a cloudy appearance, whereas in haemoglobinuria it is clear like rosé wine. Haemoglobinuria occurs in runners who have a very poor style, in particular a high, stamping gait; it also occurs when they run on hard roads as opposed to across country or on grass. There is a reason to believe that other activities which involve repetitive footstrikes such as high impact aerobics can have a similar effect. If it occurs, the exerciser should try to develop a better style. Well-cushioned shoes can also prevent the problem.

Although blood and haemoglobin loss in the urine are well documented, it is highly unlikely that they cause significant iron deficiency. A very small amount of blood can cause marked discoloration of the urine.

Blood loss from the gut during exercise and diarrhoea (often referred to as 'runner's trots') may also occur, particularly in high mileage runners or runners who have recently increased their mileage. The cause may be the cumulative effect of repeated minor trauma as the abdominal contents bounce up and down with each footstrike. Alternatively, the bowel may become more permeable or 'leaky' as it is starved of oxygen during intense exercise (the blood is diverted away from the gut to the muscles, where more blood is required). After exercise, when the blood returns to the bowel, it may pass through the more permeable bowel wall where it may cause diarrhoea due to an irritant effect. One study in which stool samples were analysed before and after a marathon showed that the amount of haemoglobin in the stools increased by 30%.

Blood loss through the digestive tract may also be increased by the use of anti-inflammatory drugs such as aspirin and many other drugs which may be taken for muscular strains. It is essential to check with your GP before taking any drugs. If they do affect iron absorption then dietary measures should be taken to compensate for this.

It has been claimed that iron deficiency is common amongst runners and is the main cause of athletes' anaemia. This is mainly as a result of finding lowered ferritin levels in athletes. Although serum ferritin is normally a good guide to iron stores, it is not reliable in runners. There are many ways to estimate iron stores, but the most accurate is from bone marrow sampling which is unpleasant at best and painful at worst.

There have been studies which analysed ferritin marrow samples for iron stores in runners and controls. One such was performed by B. Magnusson. He investigated 43 middle and long distance runners and 119 controls, and showed that the athletes had lowered haemoglobin and ferritin levels. From these results one might presume that iron stores were low and anaemia likely. However, they all had iron present in their bone marrow which means that they were *not* iron deficient. He explained the lowered ferritin levels as being due to altered red cell metabolism in runners, suggesting that more red cells are burst in circulation as a result of footstrike when running, and hence fewer appear in the stores.

Sports anaemia is in fact a very misleading term because the syndrome is not a true anaemia (in which there is inadequate haemoglobin in the body as a whole). It is rather a consequence of changes that take place as a result of training and is caused by the dilution of the red blood cells by the increased volume of plasma (the watery part of the blood) which is a beneficial adaptation to aerobic exercise. Although measures of haemoglobin and ferritin may appear lower, there is actually the same amount of these substances in total in the body – they have simply been 'watered down'. Hence sports anaemia is only perceived as a problem if haemoglobin concentration is considered in isolation. It is important to realise that this is simply one adaptation to training which results in improved delivery of oxygen to the tissues. It is clear that this gives an improved and not diminished athletic performance. So athletes who exhibit sports anaemia are not ill; conversely, they are actually coping effectively with the stresses of their training load.

This does not mean that sports anaemia and iron deficiency anaemia may not co-exist. The lowered ferritin level in runners makes iron deficiency difficult to diagnose. Every exerciser should check their dietary intake of iron. If ferritin levels and dietary levels of iron are low, supplementation with the advice of a GP may be considered.

Sports anaemia and women athletes

Even though sports anaemia is not a true indication of anaemia and iron deficiency, many studies have shown that female athletes do not consume the RNI for iron of 14.8 mg per day. Some females may even be consuming less than 10 mg per day. Many studies have also revealed inadequate calorie intake, probably as a result of a desire to lose weight; as calorie intake is reduced, so is dietary iron intake, and hence a well-intentioned desire for fitness and weight loss may inadvertently lead to reduced performance due to iron deficiency anaemia. Females on very low energy diets (1500 kcals per day) will find it extremely difficult to consume enough iron. This highlights yet another problem of dieting and very low calorie intakes.

It has been claimed that up to 80% of elite women endurance athletes are iron deficient based on the finding of the serum ferritin under 25 µg/l. This is in the author's opinion an overestimate, because sports anaemia and the dilution of normal levels of ferritin will 'mask' the true amount of iron that is stored in the body. These reports have led to concern that athletes who have no iron stores (referred to as *latent iron deficiency*) but who are not anaemic may suffer from a reduction in performance. A number of studies have investigated this claim by supplementing iron to exercisers who are anaemic and to those who have no iron stores but who are not anaemic.

It is quite clear that when athletes are genuinely anaemic (females with less than 11.5 g/dl haemoglobin), treating them with iron improves their performance. When iron is given to athletes who are not anaemic, the majority of studies have not shown any improvement. Some of the studies in which no improvement was seen have been criticised on the basis that not enough iron was given or that the iron was not given for long enough. Patients who are genuinely iron deficient are normally given ferrous sulphate (200 mg three times a day for one month). Studies that use less than this (or the equivalent in a different formulation) or which give iron for less than a month cannot claim to have given sufficient iron over a sufficient period of time to test whether the athlete was genuinely iron deficient. One extremely thorough and notable piece of research was carried out by Newhouse and colleages in Canada in 1988. They screened 155 female athletes for latent iron deficiency (defined as a haemoglobin level of greater than 12 g/dl but a serum ferritin of lower than 20). The subjects took at least 120 minutes of exercise a week and were mostly recreational runners. On average they did five workouts a week at an average of 40 minutes per workout.

Out of a total 135 female athletes they found 40 to have the criteria for latent iron deficiency. They went to great lengths to exclude anybody who had any illness likely to complicate matters and they carried out a detailed dietary survey as well. They measured fitness through a variety of tests including an anaerobic speed test and a treadmill test with a progressively increasing workload. They also had samples of the quadriceps (thigh muscle) taken through a needle biopsy in order to investigate the possible effects of tissue iron deficiency.

The volunteers were either given a total of 640 mg of ferrosulphate per day or a placebo pill. The investigators ensured that the volunteers were in fact taking their pills by counting the number of pills remaining in their bottles after four and eight weeks of study.

After taking iron or placebo for two months the subjects were all re-investigated. Those given iron showed an increase in the amount of ferritin compared with the placebo group but no increase in total haemoglobin. There were no significant differences in other measurements. The enzyme analysis of the thigh muscle showed no benefit from iron treatment. The mean power and the anaerobic speed test showed no difference in VO_2 max (maximum aerobic capacity). The authors of this study concluded that there was no increase in work capacity (which is the best correlation with athletic performance) and that if there is no anaemia, no benefit results from iron treatment.

A particularly important aspect of this work was that a placebo group was included. Some studies which have claimed a benefit from iron treatment have not compared their results with a placebo group. This in scientific terms means that the study which takes in novice recruits and gives them medication in addition to starting them on an exercise programme will almost always show very striking improvements in fitness simply because the subjects are embarking upon an exercise programme which will improve their health.

An excellent study was carried out in 1971 in Denmark by Vellar and colleagues who studied one year's student intake (at a Physical Education College) through the entire academic year from September to the completion of studies the following summer. They divided their subjects into three groups: those with low haemoglobin levels who were given iron; and those with normal levels of haemoglobin who were divided into placebo and higher supplementation groups. Amongst their measurements they looked at haemoglobin values and their VO_2 max values. As expected, those with low haemoglobin values had improved haemoglobin levels subsequent to treatment with iron. This also increased VO_2 max and endurance performance. However, this may have been a result of their serious training programme. The VO_2 max continued to improve during the entire academic year. At the end of the study all three groups showed a great increase in their VO_2 max, but the greatest increase was in the placebo group.

The study therefore showed that the most important requirement for improving endurance capacity is training. Provided that one is not anaemic, then low iron stores do not appear to be important in terms of athletic performance.

SUMMARY

♦ True iron deficiency anaemia will reduce exercise capacity and negatively affect performance.
♦ Iron supplementation in females who are anaemic will improve blood status and performance.
♦ True anaemia occurs no more frequently in exercisers than in sedentary females.
♦ True anaemia should not be confused with sports anaemia, which is more common amongst female exercise participants.
♦ Sports anaemia is characterised by apparently reduced haemoglobin levels but performance remains unaffected.
♦ Sports anaemia is mainly the result of the dilution of red blood cells (and therefore haemoglobin levels) caused by an increase in the volume of blood as a result of training.
♦ This sports anaemia masks the true iron status of an individual and sometimes leads to unnecessary iron supplementation.
♦ Sports anaemia should be viewed as a beneficial adaptation to endurance training and *not* as an illness or as disadvantageous to performance.
♦ Females with sports anaemia are unlikely to benefit from iron supplementation.

PRACTICAL POINTS

This chapter has presented the case that true anaemia is no more common amongst exercising females than their sedentary counterparts. The discovery of sports anaemia, which is more common, should not be accompanied by panic supplementation. All individuals should follow the recommendations below to ensure that their iron intake is adequate.

Dietary surveys often indicate that females are not consuming the RNI for iron. In the long term, this may put them at increased risk of developing anaemia.

- Iron-rich foods (preferably those which are easily absorbed) should be eaten regularly.
- Low calorie diets should be avoided, as should all restrictive diets which omit major food groups. Such 'fad' diets often lead to low iron intake.
- Practices which decrease iron absorption should be avoided.
- Non-meat (*non-haeme*) sources of iron should be combined with vitamin C to help improve their absorption.
- Vegetarians can obtain adequate quantities of iron from their diet, provided that they eat plenty of iron-rich foods and consider the factors which improve their absorption.
- Iron supplements are unnecessary provided that you are consuming plenty of food sources of iron (and are *not* anaemic).
- If you are unsure about your iron status then consult your GP before self-diagnosing supplements. Iron supplements can cause unpleasant side-effects.

References

L.M. Weight, P. Jacobs, T.D. Noakes, *Dietary Iron Deficiency and Sports Anaemia* (British Journal of Nutrition, 1992, Jul. 68 [1], 253–60)

I.J. Newhouse, D.B. Clement, J.E. Taunton, *The Effects of Prelatent/Latent Iron Deficiency on Physical Work Capacity* (Medicine, Science, Sports and Exercise, 1989, June 21 [3], 263-8)

E.J. Watts, *Athletes' Anaemia* (British Journal of Sports Medicine, 1989, Vol. 23, 2)

O.D. Vellar, *Physical Performance and Haematological Parameters* (Acta Medica, Scandinavia, 522 suppl. 1–40, 1971)

B. Magnusson, *Iron Metabolism and Sports Anaemia* (Acta Medica, Scandinavia, 216, 149-55, 1984)

W.J. Williams, *Haematology* (McGraw Hill, 2nd ed., 1977)

THE MENSTRUAL CYCLE, AMENORRHOEA AND BONE HEALTH

Dr Jane Wilson

Dr Jane Wilson is a clinical lecturer in rheumatology at the University of Manchester. She was the medical registrar at the British Olympic Medical Centre between 1991 and 1994 and is the Olympic canoe slalom team doctor. She has herself competed for Great Britain in canoe slalom throughout the 1980s and currently competes for Scotland.

During the last two decades it has become recognised that intensive exercise in women can lead to abnormalities in the menstrual cycle and even complete loss of periods. This may be viewed as a bonus by some athletes, but there may be both short- and long-term consequences of this condition. Runners who stop menstruating have lower bone density than their colleagues who have normal periods. In some, bone density is extremely low for their age and this has raised the concern that they may be at risk of early osteoporosis (thin bones) and fracture. There is also growing evidence that stress fractures and soft tissue injuries may be more common in such athletes. Research has helped to define some of the causes of these abnormalities, but many questions still remain.

In order to understand how abnormalities in menstruation result in low bone density, it is necessary to have some knowledge of the physiology of menstruation. This chapter explains how menstruation is controlled in the body, the types of abnormalities which occur in athletes, and factors considered important in the development of menstrual dysfunction. The relationships between bone density, exercise and menstruation are outlined and the evidence for a role of menstruation in the development of injuries is examined.

What happens during the normal menstrual cycle?

In western societies, most girls start to menstruate between the ages of 11 and 15 years, a process called *menarche*. Although menstruation may not be regular initially, the normal menstrual cycle becomes established within the first year. The interval between the first day of one period and the first day of the next is surprisingly regular at 28 days, but intervals of 25 to 33 days are also considered to be within normal limits. Blood loss occurs for between one and seven days and is usually less than 80 ml. If more than this is lost, clots or flooding may occur and the period is considered excessively heavy. Regular menstruation (10–13 cycles per year) is called *eumenorrhoea* and women with normal menstrual cycles are termed *eumenorrhoeic*.

Menstruation is the end result of a complex series of events that start in the brain (*see* fig. 1). 'Releasing hormone' (GnRH) is secreted from the hypothalamus in the brain and acts on a second region of the brain (the pituitary) causing the release of two 'stimulating hormones', *luteinising hormone* (LH) and *follicle stimulating hormone* (FSH). These two hormones help to prime the ovaries to produce an egg and then to release it on time. They also cause the ovary to produce the hormones oestrogen and progesterone which act on the womb (*uterus*) to prepare it for the fertilised egg. In addition, oestrogen acts on the hypothalamus and pituitary to control the release of FSH and LH so that the whole process is interlocked. After the release of the egg (*ovulation*) the ovary forms a 'yellow body' (*corpus luteum*) which secretes further

63

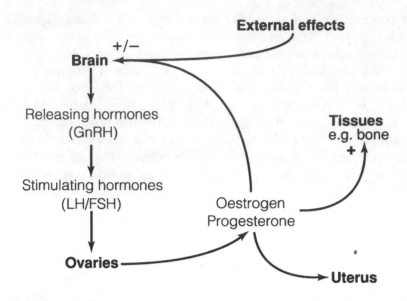

Figure 1: *The menstrual cycle*
The mechanism by which the brain controls hormone production by the
ovaries. Oestrogen and progesterone in turn act on the brain to control
their own production. External influences act on the brain to reduce the
production of the releasing hormones

GnRH = Releasing hormone
LH = Luteinising hormone
FSH = Follicle stimulating hormone

amounts of oestrogen and progesterone. If fertilisation does not
occur, the corpus luteum will die after 14 days, levels of oestrogen
and progesterone will fall (*see* fig. 2) and the lining of the womb
will be shed (menstruation). The whole cycle then restarts.

Oestrogen and progesterone levels vary by 10–fold and 20–fold
respectively during the cycle and act on other tissues as well as the
brain. Of particular importance in the context of this chapter is
their influence on bone metabolism and this will be discussed later.

What abnormalities in the menstrual cycle can occur?

The menstrual cycle is extremely complex and it is not surprising
that abnormalities occur. There are many medical causes of dis-

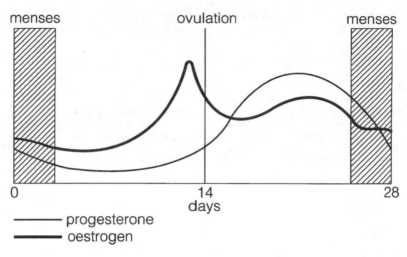

Figure 2: *Schematic representation of the changes in blood oestrogen and progesterone levels during the 28-day menstrual cycle. If the egg is not fertilised within the first few days of ovulation, the corpus luteum gradually declines and oestrogen and progesterone levels fall until at 28 days the lining of the uterus is shed (menstruation)*

ordered menstruation and these are summarised in table 1. Diagnosis of exercise-induced menstrual abnormality can only be made after medical causes have been excluded.

Delayed menarche

It has been suggested that girls who exercise intensively from a young age start having periods later than average. Certainly in sports such as gymnastics there seems to be a predominance of girls who have gone through puberty at a late age. Possibly those who exercise regularly are lighter and have less body fat than their peers; this may delay the onset of periods. One group of researchers postulated that a minimum weight was required before menstruation would start and that 17% body fat was necessary for menstruation to be maintained. Others have been unable to confirm these findings.

However, an alternative explanation is that those girls who naturally achieve puberty at a late stage are at an advantage in some sports and therefore continue to compete at a higher level for longer. To date, there are no studies which have followed large

Table 1: *Some of the causes of absent menstruation or altered cycle length. The list is not exhaustive, and if further details are required of any of the above, consultation with the medical profession is advised. The asterisk denotes conditions which are relatively common; all the others are either rare or very rare*

Absent menstruation	Altered cycle length
Pregnancy*	Thyroid disorders*
Thyroid disorders*	Eating disorders*
Eating disorders*	Polycystic ovary syndrome*
General illness*	Drugs
Post-pill amenorrhoea*	Hormonal tumours
Polycystic ovary syndrome*	
Ovarian failure, e.g. menopause*	
Removal of ovaries or uterus*	
Drugs	
Imperforate hymen	
Hormonal tumours	
Genetic abnormalities of hormone production	
Chromosomal abnormalities, e.g. Turner's syndrome	

populations of children through puberty to determine whether those who are very active do indeed start menstruating later.

Short cycles (shorter than 25 days)

Athletes, particularly runners, may have shorter menstrual cycles than normal. This is thought to be due to 'anovulatory' cycles during which an egg is not produced. The consequence of this is that the 'yellow body' is not formed and so the second half of the cycle (the luteal phase) is shorter than 14 days. These cycles are associated with lower than normal levels of oestrogen and progesterone.

Long cycles (more than 35 days)

Many athletes have periods which occur at irregular intervals, for example between five and ten weeks apart. Sometimes a period is missed because of a particularly stressful event, but in most they occur at unpredictable times. It is likely that these cycles are also anovulatory and that they are associated with low levels of sex hormones. This condition is termed *oligomenorrhoea* and is usually defined as between four and nine periods a year.

Absent cycles

Complete loss of menstruation is called *amenorrhoea* and those who do not menstruate are *amenorrhoeic*. Amenorrhoea is defined as three or fewer menstrual cycles in one year, or no menstrual cycles in six months. Blood levels of FSH, LH, oestrogen and progesterone remain at low levels throughout.

What are the causes of oligomenorrhoea in athletes?

The rate of menstrual disorders in athletes varies from 1% to more than 50%, whereas in the population as a whole it is approximately 3–5%. The condition is commoner in sports in which low weight in some way conveys an advantage to the competitor (*see* table 2). Low weight for height improves times in distance runners, and ice skaters have been shown to jump higher when they have a low weight to height ratio. In gymnastics, ballet, ice-skating and ice-dance, performance is partly judged on the aesthetic appeal of the athlete and 'thinness' may be an advantage. In this group of athletes, estimates of menstrual irregularities are nearly all greater than 25%. At risk too are the competitors who have to conform to a certain weight category. Some of these athletes may compete well below their natural weight.

These observations have focused attention on the role of weight and body composition in the development of the disorder – and indeed these appear to be key elements. Usually it is the accumulation of a number of risk factors that precipitates the change. Figure 3 shows a number of factors which appear to be related to menstrual dysfunction and some of these are discussed in more detail below. But how do these various factors cause disruption in

Table 2: *Categorisation of sports according to whether low body mass may improve performance or increase marks gained during performance*

Low weight not of specific benefit to performance	Low weight likely to improve performance	Performance judged on aesthetic appeal	Competing in weight categories
Heavy-weight rowing Ball games (e.g. lacrosse, hockey, basketball, netball, tennis) Golf Sprinting Field events (throwing) Contact sports Swimming Water polo Skiing Speed skating Luge/bobsleigh	Running (middle-distance, long-distance, ultra, X-country) Orienteering Race-walking Jumping Pole vault Rowing (cox) Jockeys (flat-racing) Cycling Triathlon Climbing (competitive) Windsurfing (Olympic) Sailing (some classes)	Gymnastics Rhythmic gymnastics Figure skating Ice dance Dancing (ballet, competitive) Bodybuilding Synchro swimming Diving	Judo Martial arts Lightweight rowing Wrestling Weight-lifting

this physiological process? Studies on the hormonal changes in athletic amenorrhoea have shown that it is at the level of the hypothalamus that the abnormalities start. By an unknown mechanism, the hypothalamus is inhibited from producing the correct amount of releasing hormone. This in return reduces the production of LH and FSH from the pituitary and so the ovary is

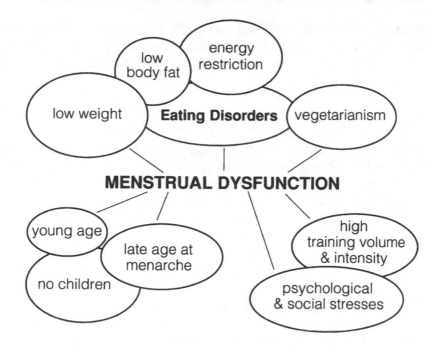

Figure 3: *Non-medical factors likely to contribute to the development of menstrual irregularity in athletes. Those women with the greatest number of risk factors are most likely to develop oligomenorrhoea*

not stimulated to prepare an egg for release. The yellow body is not formed and levels of oestrogen and progesterone remain low throughout the cycle.

Training volume

There is a strong relationship between the volume of training and the incidence of irregular periods in runners. In one study an almost linear relationship between the number of miles run per week and the prevalence of amenorrhoea was found. Approximately 28% of those running 40 miles per week had amenorrhoea, whereas nearly 45% of those running 80 miles per week were affected. In the same study sedentary women, matched for age, had only a 2% incidence of amenorrhoea. Similar values have been found by other research workers.

At present it is not known whether it is only the *volume* of training that is important or whether the *intensity* of training has an additional effect. It is also unknown whether it is possible to avoid this undesirable effect of high mileage by cross-training with cycling, swimming or other training modalities. Research is eagerly awaited in this field.

Body composition

In the study quoted above, the relationship between miles run per week and amenorrhoea held true even when the athletes were split according to weight category. However, those athletes who weighed less than 50 kg were twice as likely to be amenorrhoeic than those weighing more than 50 kg. Weight thus appears to be of great significance in this equation.

Many studies have shown that amenorrhoeic athletes weigh less, have less body fat and a lower weight for height ratio than athletes with normal cycles. Although not all researchers agree with these findings, anecdotal reports are common in which the athlete acknowledges that when her weight drops below a certain value she ceases to menstruate. The weight at which this occurs is specific for each athlete and might partially explain why not all research is in agreement on this issue.

Energy restriction and eating disorders

Most athletes do not need to diet in order to maintain optimum weight, but some pay particular attention to calorie intake and restrict food consumption to very low levels. In many, the urge to diet is based on erroneous beliefs that they are too fat. In one study of teenage American swimmers, 17.9% of underweight girls and 60.5% of average-weight girls were inappropriately trying to lose weight. Restriction of calories may be implicated in the development of amenorrhoea: analysis of ten recently published papers reveals that amenorrhoeic runners consume an average of 300 kcal per day less than eumenorrhoeic runners (1737 kcal/day^{-1} versus 2026 kcal/day^{-1}). It is tempting to suppose that there is a minimum energy intake required by the body for basic physiological functions to occur, but as yet a direct link between low energy intake and menstrual abnormality has not yet been proven.

Not only do athletes restrict calories, they may also develop full eating disorders such as anorexia nervosa and bulimia nervosa, both of which are well known to be associated with abnormal menstruation. These disorders are covered in chapter 8 and will therefore not be discussed in great depth here. A recent study carried out at the British Olympic Medical Centre on fifty national and international middle- and long-distance runners found that 50% of the amenorrhoeic athletes had either subclinical or clinical eating disorders, whereas only 12% of the eumenorrhoeic runners were affected. Similar results have been obtained by other workers in a variety of sports. A combination of psychological stresses and insufficient calorie intake can also cause menstrual disruption.

Vegetarianism

In several studies carried out on runners, a higher incidence of vegetarianism has been noted in those with irregular periods. However, all of these papers have involved very small numbers of athletes. In non-athletic women, vegetarian weight-reducing diets can induce menstrual irregularities such as loss of ovulation or amenorrhoea. This may be an area of fruitful research in the future, but at present only cautious conclusions should be drawn.

Previous menstrual history

Women who have had a late menarche or who have had previous menstrual irregularity are more likely to develop oligo- or amenorrhoea if they start to train intensively. Conversely, women seem less likely to develop irregular periods with training after they have had children. Even athletes who have had prolonged amenorrhoea prior to pregnancy may have completely regular periods afterwards, despite intensive training. This may be due to increases in weight or body fat but may also represent changes occurring at the hypothalamic level.

Psychological stress

It is well recognised that women from all walks of life can stop having periods during times of stress. In the life of a young athlete there are often many conflicting stresses such as school or college work, exams, boyfriends, qualification races and family pressures.

71

A combination of these may be sufficient to interrupt the menstrual cycle for a short time.

Can amenorrhoeic women become pregnant?

Many active women are concerned that prolonged amenorrhoea means that they are infertile. This is not the case. It is even possible to conceive a baby before having a period. This is because the ovary produces the egg when the lining of the uterus is primed and it is only if the egg is not fertilised that the lining is shed (menstruation). Therefore, be warned that contraception must still be practised!

EXERCISE, SEX HORMONES AND BONE DENSITY

How does exercise affect bone strength?

Bone is not an inert substance that, once formed, stays the same for life. Instead it is in a constant state of turnover so that old bone is removed and new bone is laid down. This enables bone to maintain its strength and to adapt to changes in its environment. In particular, bone responds to mechanical tension so that new bone is built up in places of maximum strain (for example in the legs of a runner, the forearm of a tennis player or the lumbar spine of a rower). Exercise therefore has beneficial effects on the skeleton by promoting strong bones with a higher than normal bone density.

It is not surprising then to find that bone density is higher in women who undertake regular exercise than in sedentary women of the same age. At the British Olympic Medical Centre, researchers have shown that female runners with regular periods have very much higher bone density in their hips than the average European woman, even in athletes approaching the menopause. If this increase in bone density is maintained into older age these women will be at reduced risk of osteoporosis and hip fractures.

Are sex hormones important in bone health?

In women the hormones oestrogen and progesterone act directly on bone cells to maintain the bone turnover cycle. When levels of these hormones are low (as in athletic amenorrhoea), resorption of old bone proceeds without check whilst new bone formation is reduced. The overall result is loss of bone mineral and thinning of the microscopic framework on which new bone is built.

How does bone density change with age?

Bone density increases rapidly during the pubertal years and reaches a peak at around 30 years (*see* fig. 4). From the age of about 35 years there is a gradual decline in density of 0.5–1.0% per year until the menopause. At the menopause, oestrogen and progesterone fall to very low levels and there is a rapid loss of

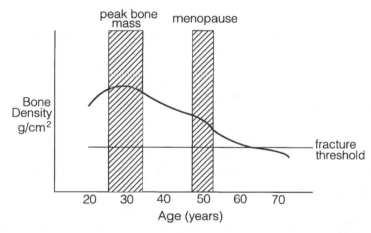

Figure 4: Schematic representation of changes in bone mineral density with age in normal women. Bone density rises rapidly through the pubertal years, reaches a peak in the third and fourth decades and then declines slowly. There is a period of 3–8 years during the menopause when bone loss is more rapid because of falling oestrogen and progesterone levels. The fracture threshold is a theoretical level below which osteoporotic fractures are likely to occur. This level is reached in the mid-sixties in the average woman. Those with above average bone density will cross the fracture threshold at a later age and those with below average bone density will be at risk before they are 60 years old

bone mineral (up to 8% per year) for several years. Gradually, bone adapts to the new levels of hormones and the rate of loss slows to about 1% per year. It is therefore after the menopause that women become at risk of osteoporosis and fractures. Sites at particular risk of fracture are the wrist, spine and hip.

Peak bone mass (i.e. the maximum achieved during a lifetime) is to some extent determined by the genetic make-up of the individual but it can be increased by regular exercise and decreased by immobility, chronic illness, smoking, some drugs and of course low levels of sex hormones. It may be possible to slow down the age-related loss of bone mineral by exercise and hormone replacement therapy. The lifetime risk of osteoporotic fracture is related to peak bone mass; the higher it is, the less likely an individual is to ever suffer from osteoporosis. In amenorrhoeic athletes the concern is that they may never achieve their maximum potential bone mass and may therefore develop osteoporosis early in life and have a greater risk of fractures.

Do amenorrhoeic women have a lower bone density?

Much of the initial work on bone mineral density (BMD) in athletes compared the lumbar spines of eumenorrhoeic and amenorrhoeic runners. It was found that BMD could be as much as 25% lower in the runners who did not have periods. However, this tells us little about how BMD in amenorrhoeic athletes compares with women who do not exercise. More recent work has shown that running has little beneficial effect on the lumbar spine in amenorrhoeic women, and so the loss in bone mineral due to low oestrogen levels is marked (*see* graph 1). In some, bone density can be as much as 30% lower than the average for their age and might be the equivalent of a 70-year-old woman. Two studies have shown a linear relationship between the number of periods per year and the bone density – the fewer the periods, the lower the density. This is also demonstrated in graph 1.

Rowers are known to have strong back muscles, and it is interesting to note that BMD of the lumbar spine in a group of elite rowers has been found to be much higher than in either a group of sedentary women or a group of elite long-distance runners. This highlights the site-specific effect of exercise on bone.

Whilst running appears to have little effect on the BMD of the

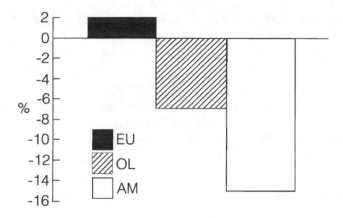

Graph 1: *Bone density of the lumbar spine of middle- and long-distance runners, aged 17–35 years, expressed as percentage of the average for an age-matched normal population. Note the linear relationship between the number of periods per year and the bone density. The bone density of eumenorrhoeic runners is not significantly different from the average population, but both oligomenorrhoeic and amenorrhoeic groups are significantly lower than expected for their age*

AM = amenorrhoeic (0–3 periods per year)
OL = oligomenorrhoeic (4–9 periods per year)
EU = eumenorrhoeic (10–13 periods per year)

(From work undertaken at the British Olympic Medical Centre)

lumbar spine, *hip* BMD has been shown to be high in eumenorrhoeic runners. Therefore, running may be a sufficient stimulus to prevent bone loss at this site. Some data suggests that there is indeed preservation of bone in the hip but researchers at the BOMC have found that amenorrhoeic athletes have considerable bone loss here despite intensive training (*see* graph 2).

What are the long-term consequences of a low bone mineral density?

Only a few studies have attempted to answer this question. It appears that if menstruation returns, or if the athlete takes oestrogen therapy, bone density increases by approximately 4–5% in the first year. It is unknown whether such an increase is sustained over the following years, but data from postmenopausal women who have been treated with hormone replacement therapy suggests that in the second year the gain is less. From the third year onwards bone density is maintained but does not increase further. An overall increase of 8–10% may therefore be expected.

But the future may not be too bleak for amenorrhoeic athletes. In one study on premenopausal veteran runners aged 40 years and over who had had menstrual irregularity in the past, BMD was found to be close to or higher than the population average for that age group. Although bone density of the lumbar spine was significantly lower than in a comparable group of veteran runners who had always had regular periods, BMD of the hip was just as high (*see* graph 3). This might mean that when menstruation

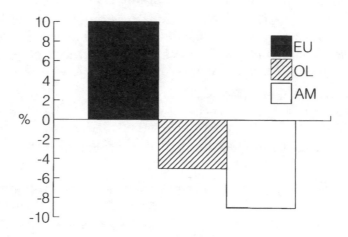

Graph 2: *Bone density of the left hip of premenopausal middle- and long-distance runners, aged 17–35 years, expressed as percentage of the average of an age-matched normal population. Note the linear relationship between the number of periods per year and the bone density. The bone density of eumenorrhoeic runners is significantly greater than the average population, and that of the amenorrhoeic group significantly lower than expected*

AM = amenorrhoeic (0–3 periods per year)
OL = oligomenorrhoeic (4–9 periods per year)
EU = eumenorrhoeic (10–13 periods per year)

(From work undertaken at the British Olympic Medical Centre)

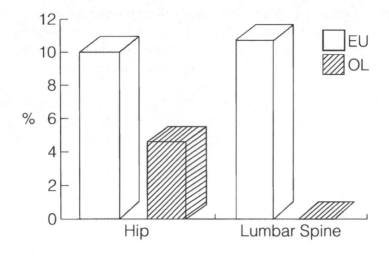

Graph 3: *Bone density of the left hip of premenopausal middle- and long-distance runners aged 40 years and over. Bone density expressed as percentage of the average for the age-matched normal population. There is a significant difference between the two groups in the BMD of the lumbar spine but not at the hip. This suggests long-term effects of menstrual irregularity on bone density which might have been partially offset by return of menstruation and continued exercise*

EU = women who had always had regular periods
OL = women who had previously had at least two years of irregular periods

(From work undertaken at the British Olympic Medical Centre)

returns, BMD increases and is then maintained because of the beneficial effects of exercise. To determine whether this applies to all women with amenorrhoea, long-term studies are required which follow women runners from their teens to the menopause at least.

Do amenorrhoeic women have more muscle and tendon injuries?

There are many anecdotal reports of runners who seem to have frequent soft tissue injuries. Many of these runners do not have regular periods. Studies on both runners and dancers have found a higher frequency of soft tissue injuries in those with irregular periods. It is unclear why this may be so, although oestrogen does have some effect on tendons and ligaments. For instance, just prior to giving birth – when oestrogen levels are very high – the mother's ligaments become supple and stretch readily. This enables the pelvis to widen to allow the birth of the child. It is possible that the opposite applies in athletes; that when oestrogen levels are very low, ligaments become less supple and more susceptible to injury.

Are stress fractures more common in women with menstrual irregularity?

Several reports have shown an increased incidence of stress fractures in athletes with menstrual irregularity. Initially it was postulated that this was due to low bone density, but subsequent studies have not confirmed this. An alternative explanation may be that adequate oestrogen levels are required for the normal bone turnover cycle. If oestrogen levels are low, bone adaptation is slowed and microfractures occur more readily or heal more slowly. Again, further research is required in this area.

The full bone turnover cycle takes about three months and major changes in training techniques should therefore be planned gradually over at least 10 weeks. If training is altered too rapidly, microscopic fractures can occur in bone; if these are not allowed to heal they can ultimately lead to a stress fracture. A typical example is that of a long-distance runner who returned to training after injury and aimed to reach her previous level of 50 miles per week within six weeks. Four to eight weeks after training started she had gradual onset of pain in her shin and a stress fracture was diagnosed.

Is there a greater risk of osteoporotic fractures?

There are several reports of stress fractures leading to complete fractures, but only recently has there been a report of an oesto-porotic-type fracture occurring in a young athlete. In the case reported, a 30-year-old long-distance runner with a history of seven years of athletic amenorrhoea was known to have bone density below the lower limit of normal for her age. She had had several stress fractures and it was while she was recovering from one of these that she slipped at the swimming-pool and fractured her upper arm. The type of fracture sustained was that commonly seen in postmenopausal women with osteoporosis.

It is perhaps surprising that more athletes with low bone density do not sustain osteoporotic fractures. It is possible that, although bone density is similar to that of older women, there is less damage to the microscopic framework. This allows the bone to withstand greater forces before fractures occur. It is also possible that, because the microscopic framework is still intact, recovery from low bone density is more likely in the young athlete compared to the 70-year-old woman. These questions have not yet been answered.

How can athletic amenorrhoea be treated?

Although many questions remain about the long-term consequences of amenorrhoea, current opinion is that it should be investigated and treated (if appropriate) when it lasts for longer than six months. General practitioners will be able to exclude many of the common causes of disordered menstruation, but full assessment and management will require referral to a specialist with an interest in this field. Such doctors may be gynaecologists, endocrinologists, bone specialists or sports physicians. Other specialists may also need to be consulted, such as sports nutritionists, exercise physiologists, psychologists and psychiatrists. Investigation will entail detailed histories, physical examination, blood tests and in some cases special scans. If amenorrhoea is prolonged it is appropriate to measure bone density of the lumbar spine and/or hip.

Treatment with hormones may not be necessary if risk factors such as low weight, eating disorders and over-training can be reduced so that menstruation is resumed. However, many athletes are unwilling to reduce training or gain weight and if amenorrhoea continues despite reduction of all other risk factors, hormone therapy is usually prescribed. Precisely which hormone preparation is used will depend on individual circumstances and the preference of the specialist. Both the oestrogen-

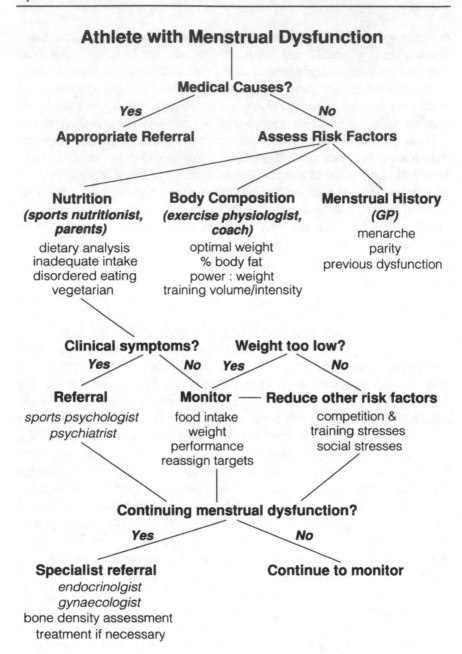

Figure 5: *Suggested flow diagram for the assessment and management of menstrual dysfunction in athletes. Specialists who may be able to provide help at each stage are shown in italics*

containing oral contraceptive pill (OCP) and hormone replacement therapy (HRT) are likely to reduce further loss of bone mineral and may slightly increase bone density.

Hormone replacement therapy is designed to replace oestrogen and progesterone in physiological amounts in postmenopausal women. The amount of each type of hormone may not therefore suit all premenopausal women, but the advantage is that they are 'natural' hormones and therefore have fewer side-effects on the blood than the OCP (the OCP contains synthetic oestrogen and progesterone in relatively large amounts; this suppresses the normal menstrual cycle by preventing the release of LH and FSH by the brain). Side-effects common to both forms of treatment include weight gain, breast tenderness, breakthrough bleeding and emotional upset, but most of these settle down after the first few months of treatment. It is important to realise that millions of women world-wide take both types of treatment without any side-effects whatsoever.

Calcium supplementation has been suggested as an alternative to hormone therapy but at the moment there is no evidence to show that it prevents the loss of bone mineral in athletic amenorrhoea. Certainly calcium supplementation *in addition to* hormone therapy is a sensible approach, particularly as the diet of some athletes is low in this essential mineral.

Hormone treatment can continue for many years until the athlete decides to reduce training or start a family. In most cases, normal menstruation returns within a matter of months. Failure to start menstruating within a year suggests that there are other causes of menstrual disorder such as a medical problem, a persistent eating disorder or low body weight. In a few women, special hormone therapy will help to 'kick-start' the system. A flow diagram for the suggested management of athletic amenorrhoea is given in fig. 5.

Case History

♦ A 14-year-old county standard runner was told by one of her 'friends' that her tummy stuck out. She decided to diet and lost half a stone. It made no difference to her shape but she ran faster. This encouraged her to lose more weight and again she ran faster. She was now 7 stone and was winning

---

races. She felt good and people were starting to talk about her. So she lost more weight. She felt guilty every time she ate so she made sure she always felt 'empty' by vomiting after meals. She weighed 6 stone.

♦ By now she was training at least twice a day and felt exhausted all the time. However, she still knew that she was fat and had to lose more weight. She developed a stress fracture.

♦ When she was 5 stone she was admitted to an adolescent psychiatric unit for management of her anorexia and bulimia. Two years later her eating habits were improving but she still had not had any periods and had had three stress fractures. She was referred to a hormone specialist who started her on treatment. One year later she had nearly conquered her eating problems, weighed 7 stone and was starting to run well again. Bone density measurements at this stage revealed to her to be 10% below average for her age.

SUMMARY

♦ Exercise increases bone mineral density (BMD). Generally, active women have a higher bone density and lower risk of osteoporosis than sedentary women.

♦ Menstrual problems such as oligomenorrhoea (irregular periods) and amenorrhoea (absent periods) are more common in women involved in sports where a low body weight and body fat are considered advantageous, for example in long distance running, gymnastics and figure skating.

♦ There is no single cause of amenorrhoea; rather a combination of factors are responsible. These include high training volume and possibly intensity, psychological stress, low body fat levels, low body weight, calorie restriction, late age at menarche and disordered eating.

♦ Subclinical and clinical eating disorders are more common among exercisers with amenorrhoea compared with those with normal periods.

- Bone mineral density is significantly lower in amenorrhoeic athletes compared with athletes with normal periods. The BMD may be up to 30% lower than average for their age, despite intense training.
- There is a linear relationship between number of periods per year and BMD – the fewer the number of periods, the lower the BMD.
- Once normal menstrual cycles return, BMD increases.
- Amenorrhoeic athletes have a greater risk of soft tissue injuries, stress fractures and early osteoporosis.
- Amenorrhoea may be reversed and normal periods established by increasing body weight, reducing training volume and intensity and ensuring normal eating patterns.
- If amenorrhoea fails to respond to the above strategy, hormone replacement therapy and oestrogen-containing oral contraceptive pills may be prescribed.

PRACTICAL POINTS

If you suffer from irregular (between four and nine periods/year) or absent periods (less than three periods/year or no periods in six months), reduce the risk of stress fractures and early osteoporosis by:

- gradually reducing training frequency, volume and intensity
- changing training programme to include more cross-training
- eating a little more to put on some weight – gradually
- not overly restricting your calorie or food intake
- consulting your doctor who will refer you to a dietitian, sports nutritionist, sports psychologist or a self help group if you suspect you may have an eating disorder
- taking steps to reduce your mental and emotional stress
- taking a temporary break from competiton to reduce the stress from a busy competitive schedule.

If menstrual irregularities continue despite your taking these measures, ask your GP to refer you to a specialist.

5

NUTRITION FOR TEAM SPORTS

John Brewer

John Brewer BSc MPhil is Head of the Human Performance Centre at Lilleshall National Sports Centre, specialising in the provision of sports science support to athletes, particularly those involved in team sports. He has worked with the England cricket team and the England football team and published a number of academic papers.

Team sports traditionally played by women include hockey, netball, lacrosse and volleyball. Because in the past far fewer team sports have been available to women than to men, the number of participants in female sports has been relatively low. However, in recent years women have become involved in many 'new' team sports – soccer, cricket and rugby, for example – which were previously regarded as male-dominated.

The introduction of National Leagues and international competitions has meant that female participation in team sports has become far more widespread both at the elite and grass-roots levels. In 1990, the first women's soccer World Cup was held in the USA, whilst in 1994 England became the winner of the second women's rugby World Cup. Since such competitions often attract a high media profile, it is inevitable that more and more women will be encouraged to participate; however, many of the governing bodies of these fledgling sports are still small and have relatively poor coach education structures, and so advice in such areas as sports nutrition is therefore relatively limited. It is absolutely essential that correct information and practical advice be given to both coaches and competitors at an early stage in order to ensure that the athletes remain healthy and the sports continue to develop successfully.

What is the link between team sports and nutrition?

In the past, considerable research has been undertaken linking correct nutritional practices with success in individual sports such as cycling, swimming and running. This has been possible because researchers have easily been able to show that, for example, high amounts of carbohydrate in the diet can lead to direct improvements in running or cycling performance. This has encouraged many competitors in both 'male' and 'female' individual sports actively to consume high-carbohydrate diets in the knowledge that their performance will be improved. Unfortunately, the link between correct nutrition and performance in team sports is much harder to demonstrate. This is because success in team sports depends on many factors, including skill, strategy (tactics) and team work, as well as fitness and diet. Because of these different factors, it is often much harder to convince coaches and competitors in team sports that correct nutrition is as important for them as it is for those involved in individual sports.

A number of recent research studies have shown that with correct nutrition higher work rates can be sustained for longer during sports such as soccer and hockey – particularly during the second half of the game – whilst recovery rates after matches are also improved. The characteristic fatigue experienced in the second half can be alleviated if the player has consumed a carbohydrate-rich diet prior to the competition. Nevertheless, it has to be accepted that correct nutrition does not guarantee success; it is *one* contributory factor which can help to improve the performance of individuals and the team as a whole.

What do players currently eat?

To date, very little research has been undertaken to assess the nutritional habits of female games players. However, in a recent study of female hockey players, it was found that their diets consisted of 54% carbohydrate, 27% fat and 15% protein. It was also found that during the playing season, energy intake appeared to be lower than energy expenditure. Somewhat alarmingly, eight out of nine players involved in the study were found to be attempting to lose weight during the playing season: the calcium and iron intakes of these players was 30% below the recommended daily intake.

In a similar study of female basketball players, energy intake values were found to be lower than estimated energy expenditure, whilst in many other sports there are reports that females appear to be maintaining high training loads on a lower calorific intake than might be expected. If this really is the case, then the athletes should be found to be losing body weight. However, several studies report that the athletes' weight generally remains stable despite the reported discrepancy in energy intake versus energy expenditure. The current scientific consensus is that there is no strange metabolic adaptation to low energy intakes, but simply that there is a tendency for female athletes to under-report their food intake! The main problem with such low-calorie diets is that they can result in a low intake of vitamins, minerals, protein and carbohydrate.

Whilst the available evidence is somewhat limited, there are clear indications that many female games players should increase their carbohydrate intake in order to sustain intensive training and competition. However, it should be recognised that some individuals will be attempting to reduce their calorific intake in order to decrease body weight, so maximum sensitivity should be used when advising female games players on their nutritional practices. Those individuals who are concerned about their body weight should be made aware that, with careful thought and planning, a high-carbohydrate diet can be consumed without any increase in total energy intake.

What are the dietary recommendations for team players?

In 1991, the International Olympic Committee (IOC) produced a series of recommendations for sports nutrition for both male and female athletes in all sports. It was suggested that the diet of an active sportswoman should consist of between 60 and 70% of total energy intake from carbohydrate, 15% of total energy intake from protein and no more than 30% of total energy intake from fat. (For practical advice on how to achieve these goals, *see* chapter 1.)

It was also suggested that – provided their food intake was sufficient in terms of both quality and quantity – there should be no need for female athletes to take vitamin or mineral supplements. In 1994, the world governing body for soccer, FIFA, accepted that the recommendations of the IOC also applied to female football players, and advised all women involved in team sports to pay particular attention to their intake of iron and calcium.

What happens if energy intake is too low?

The recommendations of the IOC only referred to an appropriate carbohydrate intake based on a percentage of total energy intake. Many researchers who have worked with female competitors in team sports have noted that a number of individuals consume diets which have a low total energy intake. For these women, even a high percentage intake of carbohydrate will still result in a low absolute carbohydrate intake. It has been concluded that low total energy intakes are often due to the fact that some females restrict their total energy intake to control body weight. This is at the expense of consuming an adequate energy intake to supply them with the fuel that they need for training and competing. In severe cases this can lead to eating disorders, menstrual dysfunction and loss of bone minerals (in particular calcium).

Eating disorders which result in bone mineral decalcification have been linked to increased incidence of stress fractures in female athletes (*see* chapter 4). Whilst it is unlikely that females involved in team sports will cover the same total distances as many female endurance athletes, the stresses and rotational forces which are experienced in many team sports do place severe demands on the bones and joints. It is therefore safe to assume that low energy intakes combined with possible disordered eating patterns could well lead to an increased risk of injuries and stress fractures in female competitors in team sports.

However, it should be pointed out that the probable incidence of eating disorders amongst team sports players is likely to be far lower than that found in individual sportswomen where body fat levels are deemed to be crucial. In team sports, a low body fat percentage is not necessarily seen as a primary factor influencing performance and therefore these individuals are probably far less likely to reduce drastically their total energy intake. Nevertheless, those involved in advising female team sport competitors about their diets should be aware of the potential existence of this problem and, indeed, take every care to ensure that their advice does not cause females to restrict their energy intake. This is a particular concern when advising on areas such as weight loss.

How much carbohydrate is recommended?

Recommendations regarding the amount of carbohydrate which female games players should consume should be based on the total energy intake of each individual. For those who consume more than 45 kcal/kg per day, a minimum of 55% of total energy intake should come from carbohydrate. However, for females who are consuming less than 45 kcal/kg per day, carbohydrate consumption should be based on a minimum of 6 g/kg per day. This ensures that those people who have a low total energy intake are at least gaining a large proportion of that energy from carbohydrate. Use either of the tables below as a rough guide for calculating how much carbohydrate you need.

Table 1: *Recommended carbohydrate consumption for female games players*

Weight (kg)	Carbohydrate (g)
50	300
60	360
70	420
80	480

Table 2: 55% of total energy intake should come from carbohydrate

Kcals	55% of energy (kcals)	Carbohydrate (g)
2000	1100	275
2500	1375	345
3000	1650	415
3500	1925	480
4000	2200	550

Long-term nutritional strategies

It is important that female games players receive nutritional advice that encompasses the whole of the 12-month competitive cycle and not just the competitive season. During the *close* or off-season period, many games players use significantly less energy due to the fact that their training load is reduced. It is therefore essential that during this phase of the season players make a conscious effort to decrease their energy intake to avoid increasing their body fat levels. This can be achieved by consuming less food in total but keeping the nutrient balance the same – i.e. still consuming plenty of carbohydrate and moderate quantities of fat, protein and alcohol, but smaller meals and snacks.

If body fat is allowed to increase during the close of the season, players are faced with the prospect of having to lose weight during the pre-season period. This can often result in extreme dieting and restricted energy intakes to levels that are below energy output during a time when training intensity is extremely high. The player will suffer from fatigue and an inability to train consistently during a period when training is essential. If the player needs to lose weight during this time, then the fat content of the diet should be reduced.

It is essential that the carbohydrate intake remain high and that the player continue to consume high-carbohydrate meals and snacks if they are to continue to train whilst losing weight. Thus it is essential that female games players adopt a nutritional strategy that covers the whole of the 12-month competitive cycle and not just the playing season.

Short-term nutritional strategies

It is vitally important to remember that a high-carbohydrate diet is needed to support training as well as matches and tournaments. Female games players must be encouraged to eat high levels of carbohydrate on a seven-day-week basis and not simply during the short-term build-up before important matches; they should be reminded that carbohydrate is the key substrate for the provision of energy. They should also be counselled on the vital role that a balanced diet can play, both with regard to the provision of energy and to the prevention and maintenance of general health and well-being.

In 'individual' sports, such as athletics, it is common for competitors to gear their training and preparation for specific *peaks* which may occur only once or twice during the competitive season. However, in team sports such as hockey, soccer and netball, matches are played at regular intervals throughout a season, often with equal importance. For example, the first match of a league season can be equally as important as the last match; if a team attempts to peak for the final of a cup competition, there is every chance that they will get knocked out in the first round. Attempting to peak for team sports therefore presents the coach and competitor with very different problems from those encountered by people involved in individual sports – they need to be able to reproduce a series of peaks at regular intervals throughout the season. A correct nutritional strategy is fundamental to achieving this.

How can the diet support regular matches?

Peaking for the next match should start immediately the previous match has been completed, and players should be encouraged to consume carbohydrate-rich foods/fluids immediately after each match. This is because the enzymes resposible for the conversion of carbohydrate into glycogen work most efficiently during the early post-exercise phase. Consuming carbohydrate in liquid or solid form soon after exercise has been shown to accelerate recovery rates and improve the ability of the competitor to train or play again within a relatively short space of time. Most players will benefit from consuming 50–100 g of carbohydrate immediately after the match and a further high-carbohydrate meal about two hours after this. Coaches should try to make carbohydrate foods available in the dressing room after a match and, for away matches, carbohydrate food should also be provided during the journey both to and from games. Table 3 (below) suggests some ideal snacks in 50 g carbohydrate portions for consumption immediately after the game. Remember that if food is not tolerated during this time, drinks which contain carbohydrate can be used instead.

Match preparation

Players should follow a carbohydrate-rich diet in the week prior to the next match, also ensuring that they maintain hydration by drinking regularly.

The pre-match meal should be high in carbohydrate and relatively low in protein, fat and fibre (unless the individual is sure that she can tolerate high-fibre foods at this time). This meal will typically be consumed 2–3 hours prior to the start of the match. Ideas for the pre-match meal are discussed in Chapter 9.

Table 3: *Post-match snacks*

The following foods/drinks contain approximately 50 g of carbohydrates:
♦ 3 medium-sized bananas
♦ 3 tablespoons raisins
♦ 1½ Pop Tarts
♦ large handful fruit pastilles/Liquorice Allsorts/American hard gums
♦ 4 large handfuls sweetened popcorn
♦ 1½ current buns
♦ banana sandwich
♦ 750 ml 'isotonic' sports drink, i.e. Isostar, Lucozade Sport
♦ 600 ml orange juice (just over a pint)

During the match

During the match, sports drinks are ideal because they meet the twin aims of supplying carbohydrates and fluid. These should preferably be consumed at frequent intervals. It is usually recommended that 300–600 ml of fluid be ingested immediately prior to the match, for two main reasons:

♦ to pre-empt sweat losses in the first half of the game
♦ because fluid is absorbed into the bloodstream more quickly if there is a greater quantity in the stomach.

Some players may not be able to tolerate a large quantity of fluid immediately before exercise. They should practise in training and aim to consume as much liquid as is comfortable prior to a match, 'topping this up' during suitable breaks in play.

At half-time players should choose sport drinks rather than tea or sliced oranges. This will ensure that they continue to replace lost fluid and provide some extra energy. Tea contains caffeine, which is a diuretic, and is therefore potentially dehydrating. Oranges contain small amounts of fluid and carbohydrate – large quantities would have to be consumed to influence fluid or carbohydrate status!

How do women fit proper nutrition into their day?

Whilst women in many countries are now beginning to compete in a wider variety of team sports, in the vast majority of cases this competition is on a part-time or amateur basis. Very rarely are females able to devote themselves to full-time training and competition. This means that their sport has to be combined with full-time occupations, and training or matches have to be fitted in during recreational time. This immediately presents problems for the preparation and consumption of meals, particularly as in the vast majority of countries it is the woman who has had to accept responsibility for the preparation and cooking of food. The tendency to miss meals or to eat in only limited amounts is therefore increased.

Females involved in team sports should be encouraged to eat small, high-carbohydrate meals at regular intervals throughout the day, especially if they are likely to experience difficulty in obtaining a main meal. Increased responsibility will rest with the partner or family of the female games player to provide suitable meals for her after she has completed her training or playing during the evenings and at weekends. In many societies this may require a change in traditional roles.

Individual preferences

A good coach of any squad should be aware that the training needs of his squad members will vary from one individual to another. The same can also be said for nutrition.

Whilst the general principles of good sports nutrition will apply to the whole squad, the coach should be aware that individuals within the squad will have their own personal tastes and preferences and that these must be considered when he is advising them on their diet. A global nutritional strategy which does not take these into account will almost certainly result in many individuals taking little or no notice of what is being said. It is therefore essential that individual consultations take place to determine the player's current nutritional habits so that subtle changes can be made wherever necessary. Simply asking each squad member to record what they are eating for a short period of time will provide the coach with a basic insight into individual dietary habits. Nevertheless, in cases where the coach does not feel able to give correct advice, assistance from appropriately qualified sports nutritionists should always be sought.

SUMMARY

♦ Female games players should be encouraged to consume a diet which contains a high proportion of carbohydrate. Recommendations for carbohydrate consumption depend on the individual's total energy intake: if this is more than 45 kcal/kg per day, then a minimum of 55% of total energy intake should come from carbohydrate. If total energy intake is less than 45 kcal/kg per day, then carbohydrate intake should be a minimum of 6 g/kg per day. (*See also* tables 1 and 2.)

- A high fluid intake should be maintained at all times.
- It is essential that female games players are encouraged to modify their energy intake to match their energy expenditure. Energy expenditure will of course change during the different phases of the season and also when activity levels are reduced for reasons such as injury or illness.
- Nutritional counselling should focus on the importance of carbohydrate to sustain training and playing, and emphasise that, through the substitution of fat for carbohydrate, it is possible to increase carbohydrate intake without increasing total energy intake.
- Due to the time constraints placed upon female games players who have to combine training and playing with other occupations, regular small meals with a high carbohydrate content are recommended.
- Vitamin supplementation should not be necessary if a person is consuming a diet of sufficient quantity, quality and variety. However, particular attention should be given to calcium and iron intake in individuals who may be at risk of having a deficiency in these areas, thus emphasising the fact that the dietary habits of all members within a squad should be looked at on an individual basis.
- Nutritional counselling should include members of the athlete's family, who will need to assist in the provision of appropriate meals.
- Those advising female team sports players on nutrition should be aware of the possible existence of, or the potential risk of inducing, disordered eating patterns.
- A correct nutritional strategy is vital if performance is to be sustained at a high level throughout the course of a season in which peaks in performance have to be achieved on a regular basis.
- In cases where the coach of a team is concerned about the nutritional practices of any of his or her squad members, assistance should always be sought from an appropriately qualified sports nutritionist.

Further reading

J. Brewer, *Nutritional Aspects of Women's Soccer*, (Journal of Sports Sciences, Vol 12, Special Issue Summer 1994)

C. Economos, S.S. Bortz, M.E. Nelson, *Nutritional Practices of Elite Athletes – Practical Recommendations*, (Sports Medicine 16 (6), 1993)

J. Nutter, *Seasonal Changes in Female Athletes' Diets*, (International Journal of Sports Nutrition, 1991, 1, 395–407)

Acknowledgement

With grateful thanks to Sarah Smith for her assistance in the preparation of this chapter.

6

BODY FAT AND WEIGHT MANAGEMENT

Professor N.C. Craig Sharp

Professor N.C. Craig Sharp BVMS MRCVS PhD FIBiol FPEA FBASES is Professor of Sports Science at Brunel University, Adjunct Professor of Sports Science at the University of Limerick and former Director of Physiological Services at the British Olympic Medical Centre. His research interests include the physiology of elite athletes and the anatomical/ physiological differences between sportsmen and women.

Our bodies are made up of a wide variety of tissues, but for most of adult life the two tissues which cause major changes in body weight are *muscle* and *fat*. To a much lesser extent, alterations in blood and bone may also cause changes in weight; blood may increase by up to 1 kg (2 lb) as one becomes aerobically fitter, and bone mass too may increase with exercise (although bone mass tends to decrease from about the age of 35 – for example, by the age of 65 a bone loss of about 10% in men, and 20% in women, has occurred). For most women, however (pregnancy apart), it is body fat rather than muscle which most influences body weight.

How does body composition change with age?

At the age of eight, girls on average have approximately 18% body fat. During and following their adolescent growth spurt, they put on more fat than boys, their body fat increasing to around 25% at the age of 17 and this may rise further in their early 20s. This fat increase at puberty, particularly around the hips and upper thighs, changes the centre of gravity of a woman's body and also of the limb segments, and therefore may adversely affect performance in certain high-skill sports such as gymnastics, diving, trampolining, dance and ice-skating. Between the ages of 30 and 60, body fat percentage in the average sedentary woman increases steadily, at a rate of 1.5 to 2% per decade.

Does body composition affect sport performance?

For *most* sports, a relatively low body fat percentage is advantageous for performance – excess fat tends to reduce speed, power and stamina. However, this is not a straightforward linear relationship, since each individual has her own optimal fat level at which she will perform at her best. Moreover, attempts to reduce body fat levels through severe dieting, purging or excessive exercise can result in depleted energy levels, depleted nutrient stores and poor bone health, all of which adversely affect performance. Therefore, it is not possible to prescribe an ideal body fat percentage for any particular sport.

In women, the lowest body fat levels are found in middle- and long-distance runners, triathletes, dancers and gymnasts (including rhythmic gymnasts), body builders, judo players (in the lower weight categories) and lightweight rowers. Body fat percentages may range from as low as 12% to around 20%. Female games players (hockey, basketball, football, lacrosse, rugby backs, etc.) and those in racket sports tend to range from 18 to 26%. Competitors in the athletic throwing events – especially in discus and shot – and rugby forwards usually vary between 25 and 32%. Perhaps the only serious sportswomen consistently above this are the long-distance sea and loch swimmers, whose additional fat acts as a vital insulator and increases buoyancy, thus aiding the mechanics of the stroke (to very good effect, as many of the long

97

distance swimming records, including seven of the 10 fastest Channel swims, are held by women).

What are the different types of fat?

Our bodies contain two main types of fat, *essential* fat and *storage* fat. Essential fat is present as a constituent of the myelin which insulates nerves, and as *packing* for vital organs (for example, the intraocular fat pad which helps seat the eye in the orbit; fat around the kidneys, liver and ovaries; some fat in the breast). Approximately 10% of the body weight of a slim woman consists of essential fat compared to only 3% in an equivalent man. This sex-specific fat is needed for normal hormonal and reproductive functioning.

Storage fat or adipose tissue is primarily a fuel store supplying fuel for energy production in cells (including, of course, muscle cells). The whole body contains enough stored fat energy on which to stay alive for many weeks – or for five to 10 days of continual exercise (depending on the duration and the intensity of the activity). In addition, muscle also has its own moderate supply of *glycogen* (the storage form of glucose), a fuel store which can last for about three hours of jogging. Fat is stored in fat cells or adipocytes. The average woman with 25 to 28% body fat has about 30 to 40 thousand million adipocytes, each containing about 45 micrograms of fat. With increasing fatness, the adipocytes may each gain up to twice this amount of fat.

The tissue known as *brown fat* is present particularly in hibernating mammals, also in babies and young children, and some persists in adults. Far from acting as an energy store, the function of this tissue is to *metabolise* fat at high rates, to generate heat, and so stop such mammals from freezing to death. It has been postulated more generally to act as a 'weight thermostat' – a 'ponderostat' – to burn off excess calories, and so possibly help to regulate weight. However, its exact role in humans is still unclear.

How important is storage fat?

Fat is used for energy during all types of aerobic activities including sitting, walking and even sleeping. When we are exercising at

Table 1: *Sex differences in percentage body fat of men and women in their 20s*

Men	Women	% Fat
Thin		7
Average		12
Plump	Thin	18
Fat	Average	26
	Plump	31
	Fat	>36

low to moderate rates of exertion, as in walking, slow jogging or slow swimming, a large proportion of the energy comes from fat. Indeed, at moderate levels of exertion such as these, fat is utilised directly from the fat depots via the blood to the muscles. It is only when the rate of exercise is increased, as in fast walking, running or swimming, that the muscles start using more glycogen (and some glucose from the blood) and less fat. During anaerobic exercise (for example sprinting and throwing), no fat is used at all.

The quantity of storage fat differs between men and women, with women generally having considerably more fat (*see* table 1, which shows the approximate body fat percentages in various categories – from thin to fat). The difference in absolute quantity of fat between the sexes amounts to just enough to make a full-term baby (60,000–80,000 kcal).

Incidentally, it is the extra fat mass which is one of the main reasons why women's running events are slightly slower than men's – about 90 to 92% as fast. However, that same fat mass helps women to resist cold in swimming, sailing, high mountain climbing and polar expeditions, and therefore provides an advantage.

Can low body fat cause amenorrhoea?

There are a number of causes of amenorrhoea or cessation of periods, including emotional or psychological stress, drug abuse, chronic illness, high volumes of strenuous training (as in endurance running, gymnastics or rowing) – and marked weight loss or fat loss. Other factors being equal, lowering body weight or body fat below individual threshold levels will trigger amenorrhoea, and subsequently increase the risk of premature bone loss, early osteoporosis and possible stress fractures in sportswomen. Studies on runners have shown that those who were significantly lighter had higher rates of amenorrhoea than their heavier counterparts on similar training and racing mileage. Also, in rowing, lightweight crews tend to have higher incidences of amenorrhoea than heavyweight crews, although they are engaged in very similar training schedules and racing programmes.

Weight and fat loss may act in two ways to produce or trigger this effect (even if it may only be the proverbial 'last straw' in a complex process). First, they may act on the great integrating brain centre, the hypothalamus, either directly or via higher nerve centres, causing it to lower its secretion of 'pituitary releasing factors'. These factors act on the main regulator of the body's hormones, the pituitary gland (sited just above the roof of your mouth), and depress its cyclic secretion of luteinising and follicle-stimulating hormones. This in turn lowers the stimulus to the ovaries, causing them to secrete less of the sex hormones which periodically affect the uterus. Second, weight loss and – perhaps particularly – fat loss may directly influence the metabolism of the ovarian hormones which affect the uterus, reducing their effect. Thus there may be a lower secretion of less effective hormones, and the uterus stops responding. These rather complex events are shown diagramatically in figure 1.

The percentage of body fat below which amenorrhoea develops varies markedly from one person to the next. It can be anywhere between 15 and 20%. Thus weight loss or a loss of fat to very low percentages may trigger amenorrhoea. Similarly, an increase of weight or fat usually induces a revival of normal periods. For more information on this, refer to chapter 4.

How can body fat be measured?

There are numerous methods of varying sophistication for measuring body fat, but determining the thickness of the skin at specific sites with callipers is the simplest and by far the most widely used method of gaining a useful estimate of body fat. The skin is itself a fat depot, and it correlates fairly well with the other

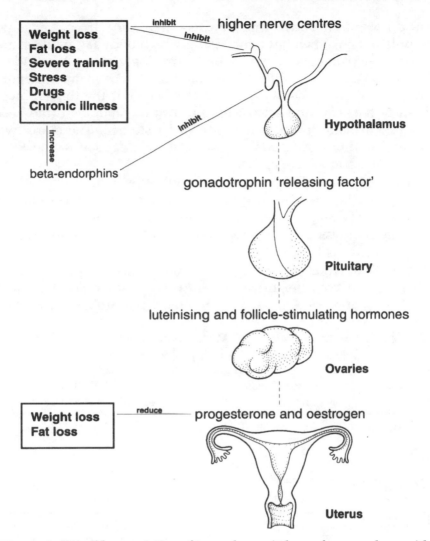

Figure 1: *Possible association of irregular periods or of amenorrhoea with weight loss or fat loss. Loss of weight or of fat may, with various other factors, act through higher nerve centres in the brain, through its hypothalamus or via endorphins to lower the secretion of 'releasing factors' from the hypothalamus which normally stimulate the pituitary to produce luteinising and follicle-stimulating hormones. Depression of these two pituitary hormones results in upset or failure of menstruation through cutting down the production of progesterone and oestrogen which prepare the uterus each month. Also, the loss of weight and fat may influence oestrogen metabolism which may also adversely affect the uterus. Note that weight and fat loss are implicated at two stages of the process*

fat depots in the body. Appearances can be very deceptive; some slim-looking women have surprisingly high body fat, while some plumper-looking women can be surprisingly muscular underneath and carry less fat than one might think. The main fat depots in women are typically (though not always) in the thighs, hips, back of the arms and bust, while in men the abdomen (the beer belly) is usually the principal site of fat storage. There are two other, less direct, methods of assessing body fat status: the *Body Mass Index* and *Waist/Hip Ratio*.[1]

The Body Mass Index (BMI) is found by weighing yourself in kilograms; then by measuring your height in meters and squaring this; then dividing the weight by this squared height. The Royal College of Physicians has prepared a table of BMI values, reproduced below as table 2.

The BMI tends to reflect body fat increases: your weight changes, but your height stays relatively constant. So, the lower one's weight becomes, the lower the BMI. The problem with BMI

Table 2: *Male and female Body Mass Index categories (n.b. not body fat %s) as defined by the Royal Society of Physicians*

Male	Body Mass Index	UK Distribution (% of National Survey)
Underweight	20 or less	4%
Acceptable	20.1–25	47%
Overweight	25.1–30	41%
Obese	Over 30	8%
Female	Body Mass Index	UK Distribution (% of National Survey)
Underweight	18.6 or less	2%
Acceptable	18.7–23.8	42%
Overweight	23.9–28.5	37%
Obese	Over 28.5	19%

[1] For detailed tables by age for both the BMI and the Waist/Hip Ratio, see Appendix A of the Allied Dunbar National Fitness Survey, published in 1992 by the Sports Council.

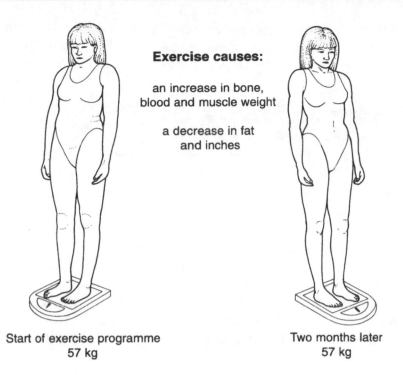

Exercise causes:

an increase in bone,
blood and muscle weight

a decrease in fat
and inches

Start of exercise programme
57 kg

Two months later
57 kg

Figure 2: *Showing that body weight may not change much in the early stages of an exercise programme, although body composition may well change appreciably*

for sportswomen is that it uses a single value for simple body mass, and no account is taken of whether this weight contains a lot of muscle or a lot of fat! Also, athletes and women on exercise programmes may lose fat and put on muscle and other tissues, so their weight may stay the same (or even increase slightly) although their body composition may have changed decidedly for the better (as shown in figure 2). However, the BMI is a useful guide in health terms for most women – and may prompt some into a health-related activity programme.

The usual threshold for defining *overweight* in women (and men) is a BMI of between 25 to 30, and for *obesity* a BMI of over 30. On this scale, nearly 53% of men and 44% of women are in the overweight or obese category. However, the Royal Society of Physicians proposed a different (harder!) scale for women (shown in table 2) whereby well over 50% of women would be classified as overweight or above. Nevertheless, in health terms –

according to major surveys correlating death risk and BMI – BMIs of between 23 and 29 for women appear to be the healthiest. It is probably worse to be much below 21 than it is to be as far above 31.

Recently, Australian researchers strongly challenged the focus of attention given to overweight women, stating that 'men and boys are at a far higher risk of the medical complications of obesity than women and girls'. Bill Tuxworth, Field Director of the National Fitness Survey, notes the paradox that 'men – who have most to fear from obesity – are under little pressure to control their weight, while women and girls, for most of whom obesity is a minor health problem, develop excessive weight preoccupations'. In Australia, well over 90% of all persons who are under treatment for obesity are female, which has led top researcher Dr Stunkard to deplore 'the strong social pressures towards thinness, which are exerted on women as early as 10 years of age'. There is a strong concern that a literal interpretation of even some of the health promotion material could induce some

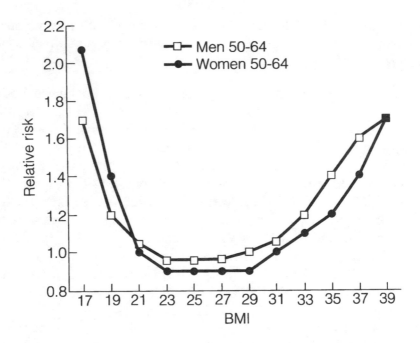

Figure 3: *Relative risk of death according to Body Mass Index*

women into over-thinness. This is dealt with in more detail in chapter 8.

If women in the upper half of the 20 to 30 BMI band find that they have suddenly put on weight over the past few months – for example, through giving up smoking, being injured or changing jobs (i.e. not through pregnancy!) – then they should seek professional help from a qualified nutritionist early on to halt the increase in body fat by an achievable, realistic combination of exercise and diet.

The other method of measuring body fat is the *Waist/Hip Ratio*, which is simply the measurement of the waist in inches or centimetres divided by that of the hips. For women, (because of their proportionately larger pelvic hip bones) it should be on or below 0.8. For men, this ratio should be less than 1.0. For example, a woman with a waist measurement of 26" (66 cm) and hips of 36" (91.4 cm), has a W/H Ratio of 26 ÷ 36 = 0.72. Similarly, in metric terms, the ratio would also be 66 ÷ 91.4 = 0.72.

The ratio is also an important health measure, although more in men than women. Excess fat in the abdomen is considered to be

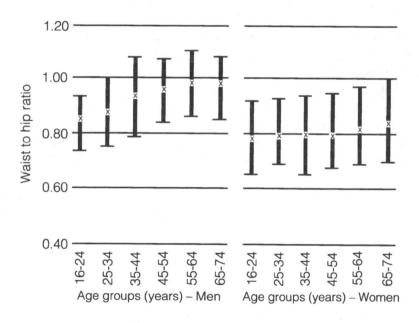

Figure 4: *Waist/Hip Ratio of men and women by age (from ADNFS). Each bar indicates the range of the majority in each age group*

more harmful than excess fat elsewhere, due to its greater correlation with heart attacks. A man with a waist of 46" (117 cm) and hips of 42" (107 cm), i.e. a ratio of 46 ÷ 42 = 1.1, has double the chance of having a heart attack than if he had a W/H Ratio of below 1.0. Women's chances of a heart attack increase to some extent if their ratio rises above 0.8, although it should be emphasised that their correlation is not nearly as clear-cut as that of men. Again, there is a greater medical risk in obese men than in women. The W/H Ratio will fall as body fat is lost, in both sexes. Figure 4 shows the W/H Ratio results from the Allied Dunbar National Fitness Survey, with the range found in each age group.

Finally, simple measurements with a tape measure may be made of upper arms, thighs, calves, bust, waist and hips circumference. These can be monitored – loss of circumference will usually denote a loss of fat (and vice-versa!). Indeed, this is one of the best measures of all!

How can I reduce body fat?

The average woman between the ages of 25 and 65 eats about 20 tons (over 20 kg) of food, yet she only gains 11 kg (24 lb) in that time. In other words, without any conscious attempt at weight control, we are regulating our weight to less than a single gram per day (less than 1/28th of an ounce). So, a very powerful regulator is at work! And it does not take much to tilt the balance one way or the other.

The important point to realise is that the body obeys the laws of thermodynamics. It neither creates nor destroys energy. Fat is an energy store. Therefore, fat accumulates if more food energy is ingested than physical and muscular energy are expended. However, if more physical and muscular energy are expended than food energy ingested, then fat diminishes.

Therefore to lose fat, one either has to eat less while maintaining the same energy output, or to exercise more while maintaining the same energy intake. In practice, it is best to do a bit of both – to expend more calories by increasing physical exercise, and to eat less energy. Exercise also has a degree of 'afterburn' effect, due to the exercise triggering an adrenaline release which may maintain a higher rate of metabolism for an hour or two after the effort – or even more following longer periods of vigorous exercise.

If a person eats 100 calories fewer each day (equivalent to two small biscuits) and expends an extra 100 calories (equivalent to 20 to 30 minutes of moderate walking) then the calorie deficit would amount to the equivalent of 8.1 kg (18 lb) of fat a year. And this is the way to think about fat loss – in the long term (up to a year), with a gradual reduction. Severe calorie restriction can depress the metabolic rate by up to 30%, and by as much as 45% on very low calorie diets; i.e. the body switches into 'starvation mode' and becomes very much more economical, hence much less food is needed. Thus what started out as a diet may turn into a relative calorie excess! Also, crash diets tend initially to empty the muscle reserves of 2 or 3 kg (4.4–6.6 lb) of glycogen – and as each kg (2.2 lb) of glycogen stores 3 kg (6.6 lb) of water with it, the 'weight loss' on a crash diet can be very dramatic indeed for the first few days due simply to glycogen and water depletion. Weight will be regained rapidly once carbohydrate intake is increased.

Diet or exercise?

Evidence is accumulating to support the suggestion that exercise may be more effective than dieting in the maintenance of a desirable body composition. For example, in one experiment three groups of people were put on a weight loss programme representing a daily deficit of 500 calories. In one group this was reached solely by eating 500 calories fewer; in the next group by 250 calories fewer in terms of food and by 250 calories more in terms of exercise; and in the third group simply by using 500 calories more per day through exercise. All three groups lost 5 kg (11 lb) over 16 weeks. But in the first group 1.1 kg (2.5 lb) of this loss was *muscle*; the second group *gained* 1 kg (2.2 lb) of muscle and lost 6 kg (13 lb) of fat; while the third group gained 2.2 kg (4.8 lb) of muscle and lost 7 kg (over a stone) of fat.

In other words, the diet-only group lost muscle and fat, the exercise-and-diet group gained some muscle and lost more fat, while the exercise-only group gained quite a lot of muscle and lost the most fat.

This illustrates the point that dieting on its own is unhealthy in that muscle is lost as well as fat – which is not the object in dieting! On the other hand, to exercise to the equivalent of 500 calories per day is too much for most people (it equals 35 minutes of squash or other equally vigorous activity, or 60 to 90 minutes of hard cycling, aerobics or similar exercise). It would be fair to say that a deficit of 500 calories of exercise per day is too hard a target to set for most people; 200 calories per day is a more realistic target. Also, it should be noted that the energy costs of activities vary according to bodyweight and to conditions (*see* tables 3 and 4 which give examples for walking).

What is the difference between fat loss and weight loss?

A combination of modest diet and modest exercise is important. Nevertheless, many people are disappointed during the early months of a programme which includes exercise because they do not lose weight very quickly – even though they may be losing *fat*. A programme which includes exercise will lead to some increase in muscle mass (not bulk), including a slightly larger glycogen store in the muscle; the blood volume will beneficially increase; and there will be some increase in tendon and bone (*see* figure 2). So loss of *fat* is not always accompanied by an equivalent loss in *weight*.

A minor spin-off of an exercise programme is that in people who are very sedentary appetite tends to 'free-wheel', whereas even modest regular exercise tends to lock appetite more into need. So when very sedentary people start a modest exercise programme they often find that they feel like eating less. In other words, they start to regain their natural appetite cues.

Table 3: *The energy expenditure in kcals per minute of people of different body weights walking at different speeds on the level*

mph	km/h	36 kg 80 lb	45 kg 100 lb	54 kg 120 lb	64 kg 140 lb	73 kg 160 lb	82 kg 180 lb	91 kg 200 lb
2	3.2	1.9	2.2	2.6	2.9	3.2	3.5	3.8
2½	4.0	2.3	2.7	3.1	3.5	3.8	4.2	4.5
3	4.8	2.7	3.1	3.6	4.0	4.4	4.8	5.3
3½	5.6	3.1	3.6	4.2	4.6	5.0	5.4	6.1
4	6.4	3.5	4.1	4.7	5.2	5.8	6.4	7.0

Table 4: *Energy costs of walking on different surfaces vary by these approximate correction factors*

Terrain	Correction factor
Road	1.0
Grass	1.1
Stubble field	1.2
Ploughed field	1.4
Firm snow	1.6
Loose sand	1.8
On level against 40 mph wind	Over 3.00

Body fat estimation, for example by skinfold measurement, should confirm the drop in fat, even though weight may not have changed much; and limb, waist and hip circumference measures should also confirm changes in contour. Also, back, thighs and arms may well feel agreeably firmer to the touch. As the programme goes on through the months, then the increase in *lean body mass* will stabilise, and weight will gradually fall as fat is lost.

What is the best form of exercise?

In exercising for fat loss, it is the *total calories* used that is the critical factor, not the intensity of the effort. For example, squash may use 15 calories per minute, so 30 minutes = 450 calories; whereas a game of golf may use only 5 calories per minute but take three hours, i.e. 180 × 5 = 900 calories. So, for *fat-losing* purposes, a game of golf is twice as good as a game of squash (although the latter's being so vigorous will promote a better 'after burner' effect).

However, regular exercise has many other health and fitness benefits. It strengthens the heart, lowers blood pressure, improves blood profile of fats, improves lung capacity, helps to prevent diabetes, improves the health of the immune system and strengthens joints. In lifestyle-related fitness it improves stamina, strength and flexibility and maintains good bone health. Also, a major benefit of exercise is that it enhances your mood and has many other psychological benefits (related to changes in brain chemistry) – indeed, it is increasingly used as a non-drug treatment of depression.

For exercise to benefit your bones – to help slow the rate of osteoporosis or thinning of bone that occurs with ageing – then the main thing is that the exercise be *weight bearing*. This gives the bone a proper stimulus. Thus brisk walking, jogging, tennis, badminton, squash, aerobics, country and disco dance are much better – for bones – than swimming and cycling.

It is, of course, particularly important to stress that fat loss should not be over done, nor over-emphasised, especially in women in the 15 to 25 year old age group in whom the risk of anorexia is greatest. It is largely fat which gives women an 'aesthetic shape', however that may be defined. Above a certain age a slightly full figure may be pleasingly accompanied by a less drawn face; and in the over-30s, a reasonable amount of fat – say 25 to 30% in women and 15 to 20% in men – is 'programmed' to be there. It is perfectly possible to be very fit and healthy, yet not to be over-thin. The skeletally-based fashion industry has no remit whatever for health! Clothes shops should perhaps stop using mannequins which, if they were real women, would often be too thin to menstruate!

SUMMARY

+ Women who take regular exercise or play sport generally have lower body fat levels (12 to 26%) than non-active women, with the lowest percentages (12 to 20%) found in middle- and long-distance runners, triathletes, gymnasts and those competing in weight-category sports.
+ Total body fat comprises essential fat (approximately 10% in women) and storage fat (approximately 16% in average women). Sex-specific essential fat is necessary for normal hormonal and menstrual functions in women.
+ Weight and fat loss to very low levels (usually < 15 to 20%) may trigger amenorrhoea and increase the risk of bone loss and stress fractures.

- Body Mass Index (BMI) and Waist to Hip (W/H) Ratio are useful health measures for most women. Skinfold thickness measurements are a simple and relatively accurate practical method for estimating body fat in exercising women.
- Body fat reduction should be gradual (1–2 lb per week or less) and achieved by a combination of diet and increased aerobic exercise.
- A fat-burning exercise programme should take account of the total calories used as well as the intensity.

PRACTICAL POINTERS

- A certain amount of body fat is functionally vital and aesthetically desirable: less is not necessarily better for performance or health.
- Decide on a realistic body composition goal that will not compromise your health or training ability. Get professional guidance.
- Use a combination of skinfold thickness measurements and circumference measurements to monitor changes in body composition – set a suitable time frame.
- Amenorrhea or menstrual irregularities may be reversed by gradual weight gain, by reducing training load or reducing psychological stress, or a combination of all three. If in doubt, consult a sports physician or a sports nutritionist.

Acknowledgements

I wish to express very grateful thanks to Bill Tuxworth, Field Director of the Allied Dunbar National Fitness Survey, for his generosity in helping with this contribution and for his splendid scientific comradeship over the past 25 years, and to John Durnin for firing my interest in body composition with his stimulating work and discussions even longer ago.

References and further reading

Allied Dunbar National Fitness Survey (Sports Council and Health Education Authority, 1992)

W. McArdle, F. Katch, V. Katch, *Exercise Physiology, Energy, Nutrition and Human Performance* (Lea and Febiger, 1991, 3rd edition)

R. Passmore, J. Durnin, *Energy, Work and Leisure* (Heinemann, 1967)

Obesity Report (Royal College of Physicians, Journal of the Royal College of Physicians 1983, 17:50:65)

N.C.C. Sharp, *Fully Fit Through Walking* (Patrick Stephens, 1988)

A.J. Stunkard, *Obesity: Risk Factors, Consequences and Control* (Medical Journal of Australia, 1988, 148: 521–528)

W. Tuxworth, *What Should Public Health Policy Be Towards 'Overweight'?* (British Nutrition Foundation, Nutrition Bulletin 1994, 19: 26–24)

H. Waaler, *Weight and Mortality; the Norwegian Experience* (Acta Medica, Scandinavia, 1984, 215, supplement 679; 1–56)

PRACTICAL WEIGHT LOSS STRATEGIES

Anita Bean, BSc

Does excess body fat affect performance?

Having a particular body fat percentage for a particular sport is regarded by many women as an increasingly important issue.

Carrying *excess* body fat is a distinct disadvantage for most sports and fitness activities. It can adversely affect your performance, reducing your power, speed and endurance. For example, in endurance sports such as long-distance running, excess fat tends to reduce running speed and induce earlier fatigue. It has been estimated that a 5% decrease in body fat in a 160 lb runner could knock 6 minutes off a marathon time. In explosive and power sports such as sprinting, long jump or volleyball, excess fat tends to reduce your mechanical efficiency and therefore reduce performance.

Can you go too low?

Obviously there is a desirable range of body fat percentages for a particular sport or fitness activity: the relationship between performance and body fat is certainly not a linear one.

One major problem is that many exercising women become

tempted to take this link between body fat/weight and performance to the extreme in the misguided belief that the lower their body fat the better.

As fat percentage decreases below a certain level this can have an adverse effect on performance. Long-term food restriction inevitably leads to depleted glycogen stores, incomplete recovery, slower tissue repair and formation, and reduced nutrient intake. The ultimate result is chronic fatigue, increased susceptibility to infections, reduced performance, over-training syndrome ('burnout') increased risk of iron deficiency anaemia and premature bone loss, and greater risk of injury.

The other major problem is the development of disordered eating patterns or subclinical and clinical eating disorders such as anorexia and bulimia nervosa. US studies suggest that around 60% of normal-weight young women have some form of disordered eating. One particular study of gymnasts carried out at the University of North Texas found that only 22% could be classified as having normal eating habits. 61% had a sub-clinical eating disorder and 16% had bulimia nervosa. Researchers agree that such eating behaviour is common among other groups of female athletes and exercisers, particularly in those who tend to have a low self-esteem. This subject of body image and dieting is dealt with in more detail in chapter 8.

What is a desirable percentage of body fat?

It is impossible to define an exact value for any particular sport. Certainly a range is acceptable, and this will depend on the individual woman. It is unlikely that any two people will have exactly the same 'optimal' body fat. For example, one swimmer may perform at her best with 16% fat while her teammate may perform equally well with 18%.

For women, 18–25% is considered desirable from a health point of view, although for competitive sportswomen the percentage is likely to be lower. One study has suggested 13–18% for women as optimal for performance in most sports requiring a lean physique. However, bear in mind that this range is not necessarily optimal for health.

Should we count calories?

Counting calories may become a thing of the past. A growing amount of research suggests that calories from carbohydrate, fat or protein are handled in quite different ways in the body and this, in turn, has an important bearing on body fat levels. Rather than simply considering overall energy balance (i.e. 'calories in' versus 'calories out'), scientists are now looking at the separate balance equations of each macronutrient. In other words, carbohydrate intake versus carbohydrate oxidation or storage; fat intake versus fat oxidation or storage, and so on.

The hypothesis that fat is more fattening calorie for calorie than carbohydrate is supported by a number of well-controlled studies. In a study of prisoners at Vermont, it was found that lean men gained weight more readily when overfed a high-fat diet than when overfed a mixed diet of carbohydrate and fat. In another recent study, men were fed 150% of their calorie requirements for two 14-day periods. In one period the excess calories came from fat; in the other the excess calories came from carbohydrate. Overfeeding fat caused much greater deposition of body fat than overfeeding carbohydrate. What's more, this effect was magnified in the men who were already obese.

Can alcohol increase body fat?

Alcohol cannot be stored in the body since it is toxic. Therefore, all alcohol ingested is broken down and ultimately converted into energy. Whilst this is happening, it supresses the oxidation of fat. So, indirectly, alcohol may affect body fat levels by channelling fat into fat storage.

Can carbohydrate increase body fat?

Carbohydrate consumed in excess of the body's immediate needs can be stored as glycogen. However, stores are relatively small (approximately 400 g) and tightly controlled. Studies have shown that when carbohydrate is overeaten, it actually increases carbohydrate oxidation. In other words, some of the excess carbohydrate is merely burned off and effectively wasted as heat! As much as one quarter of the calories from carbohydrate is converted into excess heat and the rest is preferentially converted into glycogen.

Does dietary fat increase body fat?

In sharp contrast to the other nutrients, stores of fat are extremely large (enough for the average person to jog 800 miles!). Any fat eaten that is not immediately required for energy or metabolism is stored in adipose (fat) tissue. Over-eating fat does not increase fat oxidation nor does it affect appetite. Fat oxidation is only increased when total energy demands exceed total energy intake or during aerobic exercise.

Leading researchers into obesity have proposed another physiological theory to explain why fat is easily overconsumed. Even in the short term, they say, it is not as satiating as other nutrients. Fat is not metabolised as rapidly after meals as carbohydrate or protein. While carbohydrate produces a rise in blood glucose, fat often depresses blood glucose, which means carbohydrate produces more rapid satiety than fat.

What is the secret of appetite control?

Appetite is tightly controlled by the relative amounts of carbohydrate, fat and protein we eat. Glycogen plays the biggest role in regulating hunger and appetite and therefore in achieving long-term weight management.

Fluctuations in our glycogen stores are detected by our appetite control centres and translated into feelings of hunger. So, for example, when glycogen stores are low we experience an increased appetite and have a desire to eat more. When glycogen stores are full, our appetite is reduced and we eat less. Therefore, carbohydrate balance is achieved partly through increased oxidation and partly through appetite control.

So how can carbohydrates help weight loss?

A diet high in complex carbohydrates and low in fat means it is almost impossible to overeat and gain weight. Carbohydrates have a satiating effect on our appetite while fat has practically no appetite-dampening effect at all. We could happily overeat high fat foods for days on end without any decrease in our appetite. But with high carbohydrate foods, we would feel full up much more quickly.

A recent study carried out at the Dunn Clinical Nutrition Centre has shown that volunteers allowed unlimited access to a low fat (20% calories from fat), high carbohydrate diet for seven days unwittingly lost body fat. However, when they were fed a medium fat diet (40% calories from fat) or a high fat diet (60% calories from fat) *which looked exactly the same* they overate and gained up to 0.9 kg body fat. The volunteers said they did not notice any difference in taste between the low fat and high fat diets and that their appetites were fully satisfied on both.

A series of recent experiments carried out at the Human Appetite Research Unit at Leeds University has found that when volunteers were given a high carbohydrate breakfast then allowed an unlimited amount of a snack meal $1\frac{1}{2}$ hours later, they voluntarily ate fewer calories compared with when they ate a higher fat breakfast. It was concluded that adding extra fat to the breakfast had no effect on appetite control for the rest of the day. On the other hand, adding extra carbohydrate to the breakfast reduced hunger for longer – volunteers had less desire to eat snacks later on and were unlikely to overeat during the day.

What are the dangers of strict dieting?

The main problem with cutting your calories too severely is that you will not be getting enough food to maintain your essential tissues (your organs, muscles, bones, etc.) and all your essential body processes (your breathing, digestion, blood circulation, kidney function, etc). The number of calories your body uses up at rest is described as your *Resting Metabolic Rate* (RMR). For most women the RMR is between 1200 and 1500 calories. The heavier you are and the more muscular you are, the higher your metabolic rate. So a larger person uses up more calories than a small person. An athlete uses up more calories than a sedentary person of the same weight.

If you eat less than your RMR you will encourage your body to break down protein. This will come from your muscle tissue and possibly from your organ tissue too. So you lose not only fat but also valuable lean tissue.

Remember, of course, that you will use extra calories whenever you move about, whether that's walking, shopping or exercising. So your total calorie output will be quite a bit higher than your RMR. The higher your calorie intake the greater chance you have of getting enough vitamins, minerals and protein because you are eating more food. Although it is possible to get enough vitamins and minerals from 1000 calories worth of food, for example, in practice this is quite hard to achieve. For a start, you have to eat a very wide variety of different foods and include plenty of fresh fruit and vegetables. Many exercisers with a busy lifestyle tend to rely on high fat snacks, calorie-counted, ready-made meals and other convenience foods which might be low in certain vitamins. It is all too easy to miss out on valuable nutrients like calcium, iron, vitamin E and vitamin A.

How can I reduce body fat?

The healthiest and most effective way to lose body fat is through a combination of diet and exercise.

Here is a simple eight-point plan to help you to reduce your body fat level safely and healthily without compromising your performance:

1 Goal setting

Decide on a *realistic* goal or, better still, a series of short-term goals which can definitely be achieved. Discuss this with a sports nutritionist, your coach or professional instructor, taking into account your own individual body type, shape and present training programme. Progress is best monitored by a combination of skinfold thickness measurements and circumference measurements at key sites, rather than by weighing on the scales.

2 Estimate your present calorie intake

Everyone's calorie requirements are different, depending on body weight, activity level, body composition and individual metabolism. Start with your current calorie intake by writing an accurate food diary for at least three days. Bear in mind that 1 lb of fat provides 3500 calories. So you need to create a deficit of 3500 calories over a one-week period to lose 1 lb of fat. That is equivalent to 500 per day and may be the result of eating less and exercising more.

Do not attempt to lose more than 1–2 lb a week – be patient! – otherwise your body will break down excessive muscle and organ tissue. So, if you normally eat 2500 calories a day, reduce to 2000 calories.

3 Do not eat less than your RMR

For most women, the RMR is 1200–1500 calories a day – the minimum intake required to maintain your lean body mass. Going lower than this will encourage your body to break down protein and glycogen. To get a rough idea of your own RMR, simply multiply your weight in pounds by 10. For example, if you weigh 9 stone, that's 126 lb which, multiplied by 10, gives you 1260 calories. Therefore, you would need a minimum of 1260 calories to simply survive (at rest) for one day.

4 Keep carbohydrate intake high

Aim to get at least 60% of your calories from carbohydrates. Many people cut down on high carbohydrate foods in the mistaken belief that this will help them lose weight. The problem lies *not* with carbohydrates but with fat! Carbohydrates are not 'fattening' (they contain less than half the calories of fats) and are essential for ensuring maximum fuel stores for exercise. Remember, a high carbohydrate, low fat diet makes it almost impossible to overeat and gain body fat!.

The good carbohydrate guide

- ◆ All types of bread (including multigrain, rye, soda, cracked wheat, manna bread, rolls, muffins, bagels)
- ◆ Breakfast cereals
- ◆ Dishes based on pasta, rice, oats, couscous, barley, millet
- ◆ Jacket, boiled and mashed potatoes or sweet potatoes
- ◆ Beans, lentils, peas

> * Starchy vegetables such as parsnips, yams, sweetcorn, eddoes, plantain
> * Fresh, dried and tinned fruit

5 Cut *down* on fat – but not *out*!

Since fat is the most concentrated source of calories (9 kcal/g, compared with carbohydrate and protein at 4 kcal/g), reduce your intake of high fat foods. However, do not aim to eliminate fat altogether, because a certain amount is necessary in order to obtain the essential fatty acids and help to absorb and utilise the fat-soluble vitamins. A very low fat diet, if followed for a long period of time, may lead to hormonal imbalances, lower vitamin status, dry skin, and other health problems. It will also mean a very low intake of important antioxidant nutrients such as vitamin E (which can help reduce free radical damage, heart disease risk, certain cancers and maybe slow down the ageing process). Therefore, you should include a small amount of fat- or oil-containing foods in your daily diet, preferably from vegetable sources, e.g. olive oil, sunflower oil, nuts, peanut butter, seeds.

Cut down on:	Choose instead:
• Butter, margarine and other spreading fats	• Very low fat spread; peanut butter, tahini
• Deep-fried foods	• Grilled/microwaved/boiled/baked/stir-fried foods
• Fatty meats and meat products, e.g. beef burgers, sausages	• Well-trimmed, lean cuts of meat
	• Chicken and turkey (skinned)
	• White fish or tuna in brine/water
• Pastry dishes	• Pasta and rice dishes without oily or creamy sauces
• Cakes, biscuits, puddings	• Low fat yoghurts, fromage frais
	• Rice pudding, semolina, bread and butter pudding
• Chocolate and other confectionery	• Fig rolls, garabaldi biscuits
• Crisps and snacks	• Rice cakes, oatcakes

6 Eat frequent and regular snacks/meals

Small, regular meals and snacks help keep your blood sugar and insulin levels more stable, avoiding fluctuations in your energy levels. Research has shown that this pattern of eating helps to reduce blood cholesterol levels.

Equally important, your body is then assured of a more steady supply of nutrients to replenish glycogen stores, speed up recovery between workouts and maximise your body's response to exercise (e.g. muscle tissue repair, strengthening, toning).

The healthy snack guide

+ Sandwiches, rolls, pitta, bagels with low fat fillings (e.g. banana, cottage cheese, tuna, chicken, salad)
+ Muffins, fruit buns, scones
+ Oatcakes and rice cakes with low fat toppings (e.g. banana, fruit spread)
+ Toast with honey/fruit spread/baked beans
+ Fresh fruit, e.g. bananas, apples, pears, grapes
+ Dried fruit, e.g. raisins, apricots, dates, apple rings
+ Dried fruit bars, cereal bars
+ Home-made shakes made with low fat milk, bananas and yoghurt
+ Baked potatoes with low fat fillings, e.g. fromage frais, cottage cheese, baked beans
+ Breakfast cereals with low fat milk

---

7 Eat breakfast

Skipping breakfast will not help you to lose weight. US studies have clearly shown that breakfast-skippers are more likely to be overweight than people who regularly eat breakfast. The problem with missing out on this important meal is that it increases your hunger later on, making you more likely to overeat at mealtimes or nibble on high calorie snacks. Consciously denying your hunger in the morning can also upset your body's natural appetite cues so you may lose your normal sensation and control of hunger and fullness. Again, this can cause you to overeat at mealtimes.

Eating breakfast will boost your blood sugar levels and therefore your energy levels; stimulate your metabolism and give you a significant proportion of your daily intake of vitamins, minerals, fibre and carbohydrate. It is not essential that you eat breakfast immediately after getting up if you don't feel hungry, but do make a point of eating in the early part of the morning.

The good breakfast guide

+ Porridge made with skimmed or semi skimmed milk and served with fruit
+ Wholegrain cereal such as Weetabix, bran or wheat flakes, Shredded Wheat, Shreddies, crunchy oat-based cereals (granola) and muesli; plus skimmed/semi skimmed milk
+ Bagels and muffins with honey, plus fresh fruit
+ Wholemeal toast with fruit spread, honey, marmite, peanut butter, marmalade or jam
+ Fresh fruit and dried fruit with low fat yoghurt (and nuts/ seeds if you wish)
+ Poached, boiled or scrambled egg on wholemeal toast

---

8 Avoid overeating in the evening

If you exercise in the evening, aim to consume most of your food during the daytime. Have a substantial breakfast and lunch and include regular snacks in-between. After exercise, have a high carbohydrate snack/meal (for example, jacket potato with a low fat topping), enough to start refuelling your glycogen reserves, but not so much that you feel bloated and over-full.

Try to leave at least a couple of hours after your main evening meal before going to sleep. Going to bed on a full stomach can make you feel uncomfortable and restless. If you eat a large meal before bedtime, most of the energy (calories) in the food will have to be stored rather than used for immediate energy needs. Some will be converted into glycogen (your carbohydrate store) but quite a lot may be converted into body fat.

A note on de-toxification diets

So-called *de-toxification diets* are an extreme form of dieting. They claim to eliminate toxins (poisons) from the body and 'cleanse' the system by placing a short-term and drastic restriction on the range of foods you are allowed to eat. Most comprise just a few types of food such as fruit and vegetables or fruit/vegetable juices.

There is no scientific proof for this theory, despite its fashionable image; nor is it recommended by scientifically trained doctors or nutritionists. The truth is that you will probably lose weight in the short term (mostly glycogen and water) since you end up eating fewer calories, but such diets are not a healthy nor a lasting solution to a weight problem. They should certainly not be followed for any period of time as they can cause nutritional imbalances in the body. You should aim for a long-term, balanced, healthy eating programme rather than a short-term quick-fix. **Avoid any diet that goes to extremes.**

8

BODY IMAGE AND EATING DISORDERS

Anita Bean, BSc

Most women in the western world have a distorted body image, perceiving themselves to be fatter than they really are. Many consequently spend a lifetime in pursuit of a leaner, lighter body. While some resort to the drastic measure of cosmetic surgery, most choose to focus on exercise and food intake. However, diet and exercise combined with a distorted body image can lead to an obsessive preoccupation with weight and calories, and eventually to disordered eating.

Women in the fitness or sports environment may be expected to harbour a more relaxed and positive attitude to their body image. It seems, however, that even in this context of heightened physical awareness, weight and aesthetics are becoming inextricably entwined with health, fitness and performance.

This chapter examines the influences on body image of women in general and how they respond to the pressure to be thin, and goes on to explore to what extent these attitudes are reflected in the exercise environment.

The changing shape of the ideal female form

Throughout the ages the ideal female shape has changed dramatically according to the trends of contemporary fashion. From the Reubenesque curves of the fifteenth century to the wasp waists

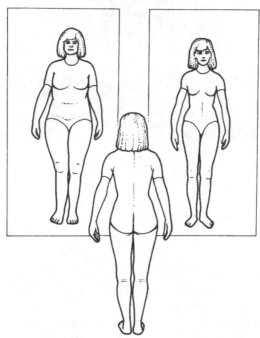

Figure 1: *Body image may be defined as the internal picture we have of our bodies.*

and emphasised posteriors of the seventeenth and nineteenth centuries, women have resorted to corsets, bustles and boning to conform to the fashionable shape. The fashion dictates of the twentieth century have, however, proven the most demanding. Women taped down their bosoms for the flapper girl flatness of the 1920s, mimicked Marilyn Monroe's curves in the 1940s, starved themselves for 60s-style androgyny, and excrcised for muscles in the fitness boom of the 1970s and 80s. Finally, the media's choice of ideal shape for the woman of the 1990s is personified by models such as Kate Moss, whose waif-like proportions (size 8 or 10 and over 5'7") promote a body shape unattainable by the majority of women.

How the changing female form has been artificially dictated by fashion trends rather than by nature is clearly shown in a study reported in the British Medical Journal, in which two Finnish doctors compared the measurements of shop window mannequins with those of the average woman. They found that the mannequins' hips were 6" smaller and their thighs 4" thinner.

125

Since World War II their proportions have shrunk dramatically by 4" around the hips and 2" around the thighs. A woman with a mannequin's body fat ratio would in fact be malnourished, weak, amenorrheic and even infertile, but a healthy body shape is all too frequently sacrificed for aesthetics in the fashion stakes.

Why should women be thin?

In the media, thinness often symbolises success, happiness and self-control, while fat on the other hand is equated with ugliness, lack of discipline and misery. In reality, many slim women will have dieted and starved, sacrificing happiness for aesthetic gain. But who is behind this media propaganda? A feminist theory is that gay fashion designers select models whose form resembles that of teenage boys. Another is that women, now increasingly competing with men on an equal basis on a business and social level, are pressurised to be thin by a male 'conspiracy' which seeks to suppress their encroachment on a male-dominated world; literally by taking up less space, women become less worthy of attention. Also, if a woman's focus is diverted to a preoccupation with her appearance, her self-confidence will be challenged and her threat lessened.

Women themselves are partly to blame for the slimming stakes. Camille Paglia, feminist and controversial author of books on women's roles and personae, believes women compete with each other to be thin, often using this as a status symbol. This competition can clearly be seen in all-female environments such as girls schools, where eating disorders can become endemic due to peer group pressure.

Do men suffer eating disorders?

For men, the pressure to be thin is less, with the media more generous in its choice of the ideal male shape. Indeed, largeness is often equated with power, strength, confidence and success – all positive male attributes. Male media attention does also still tend to concentrate on the cerebral rather than the physical.

However, fashion is now taking an increasingly strong interest in male body image, with glossy adverts for men's fragrances displaying male torsos in all their toned glory. This development may be a factor in the growth of eating disorders among men, which account for about one in ten cases of anorexia nervosa (0.2% of the male population). The true figure is probably much higher, since eating disorders are more difficult to diagnose in men and consequently go unreported. Also, as eating disorders are generally regarded as a woman's problem, men are less inclined to seek help.

In general, though, men are less likely than women to develop an eating disorder, partly because they are under less pressure to conform to a certain shape and partly because they have more lean body weight and less body fat. They are less likely to experience negative emotions about their weight or shape, and use exercise more as a means of weight control than for dieting or purging.

Do eating disorders start in childhood?

Children today are increasingly aware of body image and the pressure to conform to an ideal body shape. A study in 1993 by the Health Promotion Research Trust on 846 normal weight 11 to 18-year-olds revealed that 70% of the girls thought they were fat, with many already dedicated dieters. Researchers at the Dublin Institute of Technology in 1994 found that out of 100 11-year-olds, 44% of the girls wanted to be lighter despite the fact that most were of normal weight. In Australia too research has thrown up similarly alarming results, with 94% of school and university girls expressing a desire to be thinner, and 86% of those confessing to having dieted at least once.

It is therefore not surprising that the incidence of eating disorders among children is increasing rapidly, with the Great Ormond Street Hospital reporting a ten-fold increase in child referrals over the last ten years. Growing numbers of young girls are attending slimming clubs and clinics, although a study at Kings College found that 32% of 12 to 16-year-old girls attending these diet clubs were not overweight.

But when one considers children's role models, this situation is not surprising. The toy industry's part in developing a child's attitude to body image should not be underestimated. The association between a perfect figure, beauty and success is implanted

127

in a child's mind at an early age by dolls such as Sindy and Barbie. Relative to the measurements of the average woman, the latter's hips and waist are at least 10" smaller, the bust 8" smaller, and the inside leg 4" longer! Appealing cartoon creations such as the Little Mermaid also reinforce the attraction of this bizarre female shape.

Parents also play a vital part in shaping their children's attitudes to diet and body image. Psychologists have found that mothers with a poor self-image and a preoccupation with dieting, weight or fitness can leave a legacy of food and weight obsession to the next generation.

With fundamental role models such as these, what sort of body image is the average 10-year-old going to have?

How do women strive to achieve the 'ideal' body shape?

Dieting among women is commonplace, with a study at Nottingham University finding that six out of ten women are dieting at any one time. If diets are monitored (e.g. by a reputable slimming club) with weight loss and nutritional intake carefully observed, they can help one develop a healthier, fitter body. However, the restricting and excessive self-control practised by many dieters can give way to bouts of over-indulgence, incurring guilt pangs and warranting stricter control in the future. Inevitably the dieter will lapse again at some stage, creating the vicious circle of yo-yo dieting. Food can thus become an enemy rather than a necessary source of energy, and this distorted view can develop into disordered eating.

How common are eating disorders?

Recent figures from the Office of Health Economics show a disturbing increase in the incidence of anorexia and bulimia nervosa, with the number of sufferers doubling every decade. In the general population it is estimated that there are 125,000 bulimics and 70,000 anorexics. However, it is thought that these figures represent only the tip of the iceberg since many cases are not reported. One study found that less than one third of bulimics mentioned their eating disorder to their doctor.

Table 1: *Characteristics and warning signs of Anorexia Nervosa*

Characteristics	Warning signs
Severe weight loss	Extreme thinness and weight loss
Self-induced starvation	Excessive facial and body hair
Obsessive fear of weight gain	Claiming to be fat when thin
Feeling fat when thin	Eating very little
Low self-esteem	Great interest in food and calories
Social withdrawal	Anxiety and arguments about food
Obsessive exercise	Amenorrhoea
Distorted body image	Feeling cold/bluish extremities
	Restless/sleeping very little
	Obsessive weighing

What is anorexia nervosa?

Anorexia nervosa literally means 'loss of appetite through nervous reasons'. Typically, it begins in early adolescence but can develop at almost any age. Sufferers are in continual pursuit of a thin body and try to achieve this through self-starvation. They may begin with what appears to be a normal desire to lose weight, but as dieting continues, weight loss becomes an important achievement and they develop a more distorted body image, believing they are fat when they are severely underweight. The fear of weight gain becomes an obsession. Many take exceptional levels of exercise to burn off extra calories and avoid fatness. They find it very difficult to acknowledge they are ill and often withdraw socially, in part due to starvation and in part due to low feelings of self worth.

What causes anorexia nervosa?

There is no single cause in the development of anorexia nervosa. It is not simply a case of dieting gone awry, but can be a means through which the individual attempts to deal with difficult emotional or psychological issues. Many researchers believe that media and cultural pressures on women to be thin are major contributing factors, but also that there are strong familial characteristics. Typically, the family of an anorexic places excessive emphasis on physical appearance, a need for approval, conformity, high personal expectations, and measures self-worth and success by external standards.

What are the health consequences of anorexia nervosa?

Anorexia nervosa can have serious physical and psychological consequences. Long term food restriction inevitably results in an inadequate energy and nutrient intake. The initial signs include persistent fatigue due to depleted carbohydrate stores (glycogen). A low protein and carbohydrate intake leads to a breakdown of lean tissue (catabolism) and a decrease in tissue growth and repair (anabolism). An inadequate intake of vitamins and minerals means energy and nutrient metabolism may be compromised, e.g. low intake of B vitamins can result in chronic fatigue. Reduced iron intake will result in depletion of existing iron stores and ultimately in iron deficiency anaemia. Early symptoms include breathlessness upon mild exertion, impaired performance and lightheadedness. Aerobic capacity (VO_2 max) is also reduced by as much as 28%.

The combination of low body weight, low body fat, poor nutrition and excessive training leads to disturbances in the menstrual cycle and abnormal oestrogen metabolism. Low oestrogen levels associated with irregular or absent periods have been linked to reduced bone density and an increased risk of osteoporotic fractures.

Furthermore, anorexics often suffer gastro-intestinal symptoms such as pain, bloating, constipation and discomfort following eating. Hypotension (low blood pressure) and cardiac arrhythmias (heart beat irregularities) too are common, while more severe complications such as heart muscle atrophy (wasting), slow heart beat, abnormal liver and kidney function can also develop.

Restricted fluid intake, which leads to chronic dehydration, is often exacerbated by further fluid losses due to self-induced vomiting, laxative or diuretic abuse.

The most serious health consequence of anorexia nervosa is death, and it has been estimated by the Eating Disorders Association that over 10% of sufferers die either from the disorder or by committing suicide.

Fortunately though, many of the physical consequences of anorexia are reversible and health can be restored through a good nutrition and weight gain strategy.

The psychological consequences are, however, more difficult to tackle. Some features, such as a preoccupation with food and a distorted body image, are likely to have preceded the development of anorexia. Others, such as difficulty in concentrating, social isolation and self-centredness, are more likely to result from the disorder. Anorexia itself exacerbates low self-esteem, fear of fatness and the pursuit of thinness. There is doubt as to whether these symptoms significantly decrease even when the sufferer appears to have recovered physically. Researchers say also that the personality characteristics associated with anorexia nervosa are much more resistant to change: while the individual may change aspects of her behaviour, the basic personality tends to remain the same.

Health consequences of anorexia nervosa

♦ Reduced physical performance
♦ Decreased aerobic capacity
♦ Increased susceptibility to infections
♦ Slow recovery from injury
♦ Electrolyte imbalances
♦ Amenorrhoea
♦ Cardiac arrhythmias
♦ Increased risk of bone loss and early osteoporosis
♦ Hypotension
♦ Hypothermia
♦ Gastrointestinal problems

Psychological characteristics of anorexia nervosa

♦ Preoccupation with food
♦ Fear of fatness
♦ Distorted body image
♦ Low self-esteem

+ Depression and anxiety
+ Perfectionism
+ Obsessiveness
+ High need for approval

What is bulimia nervosa?

Bulimia nervosa is characterised by compulsive binge eating, accompanied by self-induced vomiting, periods of starvation and excessive exercise, and purging with laxatives to avoid weight gain and alleviate guilt. Bingeing is usually secretive and pre-planned and this is followed by enormous guilt and depression. Sufferers may consume up to 5000 kcal or more during one binge.

Table 2: *Characteristics and warning signs of bulimia nervosa*

Characteristics of bulimia nervosa	Warning signs of bulimia nervosa
Bingeing on large amounts of food	Tooth decay/enamel erosion
Guilt and remorse after bingeing	Puffy face
Purging – vomiting/laxative abuse	Normal weight or weight fluctuations
Starvation	Frequent weighing
Excessive exercise	Disappearing after meals to get rid of food
Distorted body image	Secretive eating
Obsession with food and weight	Menstrual disturbances

What causes bulimia nervosa?

The disorder is likely to be triggered by a variety of difficult circumstances. It has been suggested that bulimics are predisposed to depression and that this can be exacerbated by a chaotic and conflicting family environment, a confused social role and sometimes by sexual abuse. These factors lead to low self-esteem and an inability to face conflict or emotions. As with anorexia, media and cultural pressures to be thin also play a role and the bulimic sees weight loss as a solution to her problems. Her ability to 'cheat nature' by regulating her body shape by binge eating and purging allows her a measure of control over emotional confusion; they provide a temporary distraction for the sufferer from the real problem at hand. Emotions are thus suppressed and anxiety built up, to be released (at least partly) through bingeing and purging. A vicious circle ensues, where bingeing and purging become a way to remove the guilt and shame associated with the acts as well as a way to avoid weight gain.

What are the health consequences of bulimia nervosa?

Most of the health consequences of bulimia nervosa are due to the bingeing and purging rather than from starvation, as in the case of anorexia nervosa. Menstrual irregularities are very common even when the individual's weight is normal. Amenorrhoea is less likely than in anorexia nervosa.

Dental problems occur in bulimics who vomit due to the action of the stomach acid, resulting in gum disease and erosion of tooth enamel. Gastrointestinal problems from vomiting or laxative abuse may include abdominal cramps, constipation, diarrhoea and, in extreme cases, ulceration and perforation of the oesophagus or stomach rupture.

Purging can result in dehydration and electrolyte imbalances, which in turn affect cardiovascular and renal functions. Other consequences include hypotension, lightheadedness and poor circulation.

Fortunately, many of the health consequences of bulimia nervosa (except tooth erosion) can eventually be reversed with a healthy nutritional programme.

As with anorexia nervosa, many of the psychological characteristics precede or are exacerbated by the development of the disorder. These include a low self-esteem, anxiety, depression, anger, a high need for approval and mood swings. Most of these symptoms worsen with the severity and continuation of the disorder, and a vicious circle develops as the bulimic symptoms make the sufferer feel even worse.

Health consequences of bulimia nervosa
+ Menstrual irregularities
+ Enamel erosion and gum disease
+ Gastrointestinal problems
+ Bowel problems
+ Dehydration
+ Electrolyte imbalances
+ Cardiovascular complications
+ Hypotension

Psychological symptoms of bulimia nervosa
+ Food preoccupation
+ Desire for thinness
+ Low self-esteem
+ Impulsiveness
+ Depression, anxiety, anger
+ Body dissatisfaction
+ High need for approval
+ Abnormal eating behaviour

What is disordered eating?

Although disordered eating is not a clinical eating disorder as it does not meet the American Psychiatric Association's (APA) official criteria for anorexia nervosa or bulimia nervosa, it does include some but not all of the major symptoms of those diseases.

What are the symptoms of disordered eating?

Sufferers have an intense fear of gaining weight or becoming fat even though their weight is normal or (as is often the case) below normal. They are totally preoccupied with food and calories, having a fixation about their weight and a distorted body image. They attempt to lose weight by strict dieting, usually below 1200 kcal a day, and exercise excessively. They have chaotic eating patterns and often have irregular or absent periods. Bingeing and purging are common, although the actual amount eaten during a 'binge' is not that much greater than a normal-sized meal: the sufferer simply perceives it to be excessive.

> ### Health consequences of disordered eating
> - Low energy levels
> - Extreme fatigue
> - Reduced performance
> - Decreased aerobic capacity
> - Increased susceptibility to infections
> - Slow or poor recovery from injury
> - Electrolyte imbalances
> - Menstrual irregularities
> - Amenorrhoea
> - Cardiovascular changes
> - Increased risk of bone loss and early osteoporosis
> - Depression

How common are eating disorders among female exercisers?

We have seen how the pressure to be thin affects women in general. To what extent is this situation reflected in the sports and fitness environment, where performance and physical achievement might be considered paramount?

Disordered eating is so rife among female athletes and fitness participants that the term *anorexia athletica* is now applied in this respect. The extent of the problem is perhaps less surprising when one analyses the shared psychological characteristics of indivi-

135

duals at risk of developing eating disorders and those of elite athletes: competitiveness, perfectionism, compulsiveness and a high degree of self-motivation are typical traits of both 'personalities'.

Sport and exercise give the athlete a sense of achievement and control over her body. While in a confident, objective athlete this may be gained through the knowledge she is in peak physical condition through balancing her diet with the energy needs of her training programme, for an athlete suffering from or predisposed to disordered eating, sports or fitness programmes can provide another means by which to lose weight or body fat.

The prevalence of disordered eating in the sports and fitness environment is therefore not surprising.

The eating disorders 'personality'
- Obsessive
- Compulsive
- Perfectionist
- Self-motivated
- Competitive

'Personality' of elite athletes
- dissatisfied with body shape
- poor self image
- unhappy about appearance
- distorted perception of body size
- more self critical
- more emotionally reactive

Which sports are particular cause for concern?

The incidence of eating disorders is particularly high in thinness-demand sports, where competition is fierce and where the sports environment (coaches/peers) and society exert pressure to conform to a certain body shape. While leanness can be a factor in improving performance in these areas, aesthetics are often seen as a higher priority in restricting calorie intake. Gymnasts, ballet dancers, figure skaters and long distance runners are thus more prone to a distorted body image and eating disorders than women in sports where appearance is less important, e.g. hockey, netball and football.

Researchers at the University of North Texas conducted a survey of college gymnasts, with alarming results. Of the 215 gymnasts who completed detailed questionnaires, only 22% could be classified as having normal eating habits. 61% had a sub-clinical eating disorder, and 16% had bulimia nervosa. The incidence of eating disorders among ballet dancers is notoriously high. A study at Wolverhampton University found that two thirds of ballet dancers were underweight with a Body Mass Index (BMI) below 20 (the normal range being 20–25).

This pattern is echoed, though to a lesser degree, in the male sports environment. Those areas considered most at risk include weight-category sports like wrestling, those where weight affects performance such as long distance running or racing for jockeys, and aesthetic sports such as bodybuilding.

Do certain sports attract women with an eating disorder?

The training programmes of certain sports attract women who would normally use excessive exercise as a means of losing or controlling weight. The positive relationship between leanness and performance in these areas legitimises the athlete's pursuit of thinness, so that the sport provides an ideal camouflage for an athlete's illness, serving as a socially acceptable excuse to family and friends.

Long distance running is particularly appealing in this respect. Indeed, a recent survey of more than 4000 recreational runners found that 24% of the women had attitudes suggestive of a serious eating disorder.

Do certain sports cause eating disorders?

Researchers have looked at the possibility that the strenuous exercise regimes and restrictive diets required of certain sports can actually initiate anorexia nervosa. By suppressing the appetite and thereby decreasing food intake and body weight, the desire to exercise is increased. However, this theory assumes exercise as the focal point for the anorexia, whereas this is in fact often preceded by dietary restriction and weight loss. It also fails to explain bulimia nervosa.

What effect does an eating disorder have on an athlete's performance?

Long term food restriction can have serious physical consequences. Physical activity will feel harder, fatigue occurs more readily, and performance will be reduced. Recovery between training will be incomplete, and chronic fatigue (or 'burnout'/overtraining) develops. The aerobic capacity (VO_2 max) will be dramatically reduced by as much as 28% within two months of severe dieting, thereby cancelling out any performance 'advantage' of a reduced body weight. An unbalanced diet can also result in low oestrogen levels, increasing the risk of osteoporotic fractures. Indeed, the British Olympic Medical Centre has recently reported a true osteoporotic fracture in a 30-year-old.

All the physical consequences of eating disorders examined on pages 130–5 combine to hinder performance and to reduce drastically the benefits of a training programme.

How does a sportswoman with an eating disorder continue training?

It seems an extraordinary paradox that many sufferers continue to exercise and compete despite consuming far fewer calories than they expend. A number of studies, mainly on runners, have demonstrated large imbalances between energy intake and expenditure. Many competitive runners, for example, consume as few as 1400–1600 kcal per day, barely enough to maintain their basal metabolic rate, let alone to support their rigorous training. In one study of marathon runners who averaged 45 training miles per week, energy expenditure exceeded energy intake by more than 645 kcal, yet their weights remained stable. Undoubtedly, a combination of psychological and physiological factors are involved.

On the physiological side, it has been suggested that the body adapts to the combination of excessive exercise and long term restriction of calorie intake by becoming more energy efficient and reducing its metabolic activity. This would allow the athlete to train and to maintain energy balance and body weight on fewer calories than would be expected. Studies on non-athletes have shown that calorie restriction can lower basal metabolic rate by 10–30%. However, researchers have so far failed to agree on the combined effect of chronic dieting and exercise; some believe exercise prevents a drop in the metabolic rate while others suggest that excessive exercise during dieting may slow it down.

To overcome physical and emotional fatigue, many anorexics and bulimics use stimulants such as caffeinated drinks (e.g. strong coffee and 'diet' cola) to give them energy. While this may initially boost performance, the effects will not last long as depleted glycogen and nutrient stores will inevitably take their toll.

On the psychological side, the traits typical of the eating disorder 'personality' (competitiveness, perfectionism, self-motivation, etc.) combine to lend the sufferer the impetus and strength to continue training, aided by the development of great stamina required to overcome the physical weaknesses incurred from restricted calorie intake.

Despite these physiological and psychological compromises, optimal performance cannot be sustained indefinitely. As glycogen and nutrient stores become chronically depleted, the athlete's health will suffer. Maximal oxygen consumption decreases, chronic fatigue sets in and the athlete becomes more susceptible to injury and infection.

Some scientists do believe, however, that many female athletes under-report their food intake and actually eat more than they admit. For example, a study at Indiana University on nine highly-trained cross-country runners found that they were eating, on average, 2100 kcal per day while their predicted energy expenditure was 3000 kcal. After analysing the results of the Food Attitude Questionnaire, the researchers concluded that many had a poor body image and had inaccurately reported what they ate during the study.

How should I approach someone suspected of having an eating disorder?

Approaching someone you suspect of having an eating disorder requires great care and sensitivity. Sufferers are likely to deny that they have a problem (anorexics often refuse to believe that they have a problem anyway). They may feel embarrassed and their self-esteem threatened. Most fear that by admitting their problem they will be forced to gain weight or prevented from training or competing. Thus it is vital to avoid direct confrontation about eating behaviour or physical symptoms. The best person to approach the suspected sufferer is obviously someone with whom she has a close and trusting relationship.

The best strategy is usually to ask the sufferer how she feels and to let her know that you genuinely care. Be tactful and tread very gently. This may take several conversations over a long period of time. Do not suddenly present 'evidence' such as observed weight loss, starving, bingeing or purging, and avoid accusations or trying to 'catch her out' to prove your case. This will make her feel even more defensive and threatened, and will ultimately drive her further away from help.

What should I do if the sufferer admits she has a problem?

Getting the sufferer to admit to having an eating problem is a significant accomplishment in itself. Suggest to her that it would be best to have an initial consultation with an eating disorders specialist. Help her make arrangements for a consultation as soon as possible before she changes her mind.

Various forms of professional help are available. Some individuals may feel less threatened by talking to trained counsellors from a self-help organisation or private eating disorders clinic. A list of self-help organisations is given below. Others may feel comfortable with a GP's referral which usually involves treatment within a multidisciplinary team of psychologists and dietitians.

What should I do if the sufferer refuses to admit a problem?

If the sufferer initially denies she has a problem, leave the subject for a short while (e.g. 2–3 weeks) before approaching it again. Don't push too hard to start with. Repeated attemps may well be necessary, but avoid undue coersion. However, if she continues to deny the problem or refuse help and there is genuine concern for her health, a slightly more direct approach may be necessary. For example, ask her how much weight she has lost and then give tactful information about a healthy weight for her sport. Ask about her menstrual cycle, whether she feels fatigued, depressed or irritable. Once she admits to any of these symptoms, carefully ask about her eating habits and let her know that you are concerned. Only as a very last resort, where there is great concern about her health, should you insist on a consultation with a GP or specialist.

What type of treatment can the sufferer expect?

Different types of treatment are available, depending on the type and severity of the disorder and also on the sufferer herself. Bulimia nervosa is usually treated on an outpatient basis whereas anorexia nervosa can involve a period of in-patient treatment as well.

The ultimate goal of treatment is to normalise weight and eating behaviour, and to deal with the psychological issues that lie behind the eating disorder. The treatment for an anorexic patient involves restoring normal weight and health, as well as solving the problems which led to the initial development of the disorder. The treatment for a bulimic patient involves breaking the binge-purge cycle and developing a normal eating pattern.

Sufferers may receive individual psychotherapy with a qualified therapist who will determine the exact nature of the eating problem and develop an individual strategy for change. For anorexics, psychological changes often take years and require a great deal of honesty, trust and sincerity. It may take many months before an anorexic patient will start to accept treatment, gain weight and eat more.

For bulimics, therapy usually lasts for about 20 sessions over

4–5 months. The first stage, which lasts about a month, involves establishing control over eating. The second stage, lasting about two months, involves changing the patient's attitude towards diet, eating behaviour and body shape, and increasing self-esteem. After this a maintenance plan is made.

She may decide to join a self-help or support group which will provide help from a therapist but also allow her to discuss her problem with and obtain support from fellow sufferers.

Sometimes family therapy is used, particularly for anorexic patients whose disorder developed before the age of 19. All of the family members are involved in the treatment. Here, the aim is to explore family relationships, dynamics and issues which may have contributed to the eating disorder, and then to develop a family-based strategy to overcome the problem. This may be used in conjunction with in-patient behavioural therapy. Here, access to pleasurable activities or possessions is granted upon weight gain.

The sufferer may be referred to a nutritionist or dietitian for nutritional counselling at some point in her treatment. Although the sufferer often believes herself to be knowledgeable about food and eating behaviour, she may actually have many misconceptions. The nutritionist or dietitian will be able to provide correct information and work out a nutritional programme suited to the individual. She will provide reassurance about weight gain, encourage the recovering patient to eat in a variety of different settings, and can also counsel other members of the family about nutrition and eating habits.

Have you got an eating problem?

This questionnaire is not intended as a diagnostic method for eating problems nor as a sustitute for a full diagnosis by an eating disorders specialist.

- Do you exercise *specifically* to lose weight or fat?
- Do you worry about or dislike your body shape?
- Do you often 'feel fat' one day and 'thin' the next?
- Do your friends/family insist that you are slim while you feel fat?
- Do you feel guilty after eating a high calorie or high fat meal?
- Do you constantly scrutinise food labels to check the nutritional content?

◆ Do you avoid certain foods even though you want to eat them?

◆ Do you feel stressed or guilty if your normal diet or exercise routine are interrupted?

◆ Do you often decline invitations to meals and social occasions involving food in case you might have to eat something fattening?

Learning to break the habit

This guide is not intended as a treatment for an eating disorder. Treatment should always be sought from an eating disorders specialist.

◆ Learn to accept and like your body's shape – emphasise your good points.

◆ Realise that reducing your body fat will not solve deep rooted problems or an emotional crisis.

◆ Don't set rigid eating rules for yourself and feel guilty when you break them.

◆ Don't ban any foods or feel guilty about eating anything.

◆ Establish a sensible healthy eating pattern rather than a strict diet.

◆ Listen to your natural appetite cues – learn to eat when you are hungry.

◆ If you do overeat, don't try to 'pay for it' later by starving yourself.

◆ Enjoy your exercise or sport for its own sake: have fun instead of enduring torture to lose body fat.

SUMMARY

◆ Women generally have a more negative body image than men. They frequently over-estimate their body size, are preoccupied with their weight, tend to aspire to unrealistic goals for weight loss and are more likely than men to engage in destructive behaviour to attain their ideal weight.

- The fitness and sports environment puts women under great pressure to attain a low body weight and low body fat percentage. Those in 'thinness demand' and weight category sports tend to have a poorer body image.
- Body dissatisfaction and preoccupation with size and shape often begins in adolescence and may be exacerbated by a number of other factors: mothers who themselves have a negative body image; peer group pressure; perfectionist personality; media images of thinness; and pressure from coaches.
- The desire to look lean or thin often exceeds the desire to win or train well. Many women take on excessive amounts of exercise in order to pursue their obsession with weight loss.
- The athletic 'personality' is often very similar to the eating disorder 'personality': obsessive, compulsive, perfectionist, and self-motivated.
- Women participating in fitness programmes and sports are more likely to have a disordered pattern of eating than non-exercisers; it has been estimated that up to 60% have symptoms of a sub-clinical eating disorder.
- Anorexia nervosa is characterised by extreme thinness, self-induced starvation and weight loss, an intense fear of weight gain, feeling fat when thin, and amenorrhoea.
- Bulimia nervosa is characterised by over-concern with body shape and weight, frequent bingeing followed by guilt pangs, purging, starvation or excessive exercise.
- Disordered eating is characterised by an intense fear of gaining weight or becoming fat (though the sufferer's weight may be within or below the normal range), distorted body image, excessive exercise for weight control, chaotic eating patterns and a fixation with food and weight.
- Eating disorders and disordered eating patterns are more common in women involved in sports or activities requiring a very lean physique.
- It is unlikely that exercise itself causes eating disorders. Some women with a tendency to eating disorders are attracted to certain sports and exercise programmes and this environment may trigger off the underlying disorder.

PRACTICAL POINTS

- Women should be encouraged to accept the fact that their natural basic shape cannot be changed by dieting or exercising.
- Less pressure to be thin should be placed on women by the media, the fashion industry, sports coaches and judges.
- The physiological and psychological dangers of food restriction, dieting and excessive exercise are not given enough attention: these should be highlighted more in the media, in clubs and through instructor/coach education.
- Women should not feel guilty about eating anything or 'ban' any food from their diet. More emphasis should be placed on the enjoyment of eating so women can develop a healthy attitude towards food.
- Approaching someone with an eating disorder requires great care and sensitivity, and any direct confrontation about her symptoms or eating behaviour should be avoided.
- If a sufferer admits to her problem, professional help should be sought from an eating disorders specialist. This is available from trained counsellors and self-help organisations or via a GP's referral.

Useful organisations

Eating Disorders Association, Sackville Place, 44–48 Magdalen Street, Norfolk NR3 1JU. Tel: 01603 621414

National Centre for Eating Disorders, 54 New Road, Esher, Surrey. Tel: 01372 469493

Maisner Centre for Eating Disorders, PO Box 464, Hove, East Sussex, BN3 2BN. Tel: 01273 729818

British Association for Counselling, 1 Regent Place, Rugby, Warwickshire CV21 2PJ. Tel: 01788 578328

References

T.A. Petrie, *Disordered Eating in Female Collegiate Gymnasts: Prevalence and Personality/Attitudinal Correlates* (Journal of Sport and Exercise Psychology, 15, 424–436, 1993)

K.A. Beals, M.M. Manore, *The Prevalence and Consequences of Subclinical Eating Disorders in Female Athletes* (International Journal of Sports Nutrition, 4, 175–195, 1994)

J. Sundgot-Bergon, *Eating Disorders in Female Athletes* (Sports Medicine, 17 (3), 176–188, 1994)

C. Davies, *Body Image, Dieting Behaviours and Personality Factors: A Study of High Performance Female Athletes* (International Journal of Sports Psychology, 23, 179–192, 1993)

T.A. Petrie, S. Stoever, *The Incidence of Bulimia Nervosa and Pathogenic Weight Control Behaviours in Female Collegiate Gymnasts* (res Quarterly Exercise Sport, 64 (2), 238–241, 1993)

H. Saul, *Dying Swans?* (New Scientist, January 1994)

B. Dolan, I. Gitzinger, *Why Women? Gender Issues and Eating Disorders* (Athlone Press, 1994)

R.A. Thompson, R. Tattner Sherman, *Helping Athletes with Eating Disorders* (Human Kinetics Publishers, 1993)

R. West, *Eating Disorders: Anorexia Nervosa and Bulimia Nervosa* (Office of Health Economics, 1994)

T. Sanders, P. Bazalgette, *You Don't Have to Diet!* (Bantam Press, 1994)

COMPETITION PREPARATION: A PRACTICAL GUIDE

Peggy Wellington,

BSc (Hons), MPhil

Peggy Wellington BSc MPhil is a freelance sports nutritionist currently working as the nutrition consultant to the Amateur Swimming Association and national speed and figure skating squads, and is a member of the British Olympic Association's Nutrition Steering Group. She was a nutrition adviser at the 1992 Barcelona Olympic Games, 1994 Commonwealth Games and 1993 World Athletic Championships as well as numerous other international events. Co-director of P & A Sports Nutrition, she presents courses and seminars nationwide. A former track and field competitor, Peggy is in training to complete her first marathon.

The Chinese are said to drink caterpillar tea and turtle blood, the Kenyans prefer cow's blood. Countless athletes have devised their own special formulae to give them that ever-elusive 'edge' over their opponents. There are endless stories of pre-event eating practices ranging from the extreme to the bizarre to the downright ridiculous! Tales of sprinters 'carbo-loading' for extra energy, judo players starving themselves to shed those last few pounds and swimmers tucking into curry and chips (because they swam fast last time they ate this meal) are not uncommon. Myths and misconceptions abound and everyone has a horror story to tell when it comes to the competition diet. The end result is that many exercisers are left confused about the ideal preparation for their particular activity.

This chapter will evaluate the whole of the competition period by assessing the latest scientific recommendations and translating these into practical advice. Whilst it will concentrate on the physical aspects of preparation, the psychological implications of different eating patterns and food choices are also essential and should be considered at all times.

An athlete's preparation is not complete until she has considered the effects of her eating plan on the psychological and physical demands of her event. Whilst the basic nutritional principles for male and female exercisers are essentially the same with regard to competition preparation, it is vital to consider event management so that women are fully aware of the importance of nutrition over the competition period.

What should I eat during the week(s) prior to an event?

Your preparation will be dictated by the kind of event that you are competing in, the importance of the event and the frequency of competition. If you are performing a one-off sprint lasting only a few seconds, then dietary manipulation will have a limited effect. However, most competitions involve heats and finals or several rounds of competition on the same day. Fatigue in such events may be caused by glycogen depletion and/or dehydration. If you are participating in events involving prolonged, continuous exercise (for example running, triathlon or cycling) or multiple bouts of high-intensity activity (for example swimming, hockey, football, squash or tennis), then nutritional guidance may be crucial to your preparation.

Women competitors should aim to achieve the following nutrition goals:

♦ to ensure that liver and muscle glycogen stores are full

♦ to be well hydrated
♦ to avoid any new or unfamiliar practices that might negatively affect performance
♦ to 'make weight' in sports such as judo and rowing without compromising performance
♦ to plan a nutrition strategy for the whole competition period – and to be prepared to pack an 'emergency food bag'!

How can liver and muscle glycogen stores be optimally filled?

An adequate taper (rest) in conjunction with a high-carbohydrate diet will ensure that glycogen stores are fully replenished. Generally 24–48 hours of rest and a high-carbohydrate diet will allow adequate refuelling. However, the presence of muscle damage will delay this process. Training which may cause muscle fibre damage should either be scheduled earlier in the week to allow for recovery or be avoided altogether. Such training includes eccentric weight work, plyometric types of activity and hard running or body contact sessions.

If competitions occur several times a week, as is the case in league hockey, netball and football, it may not be possible to rest for 48 hours prior to each event. Such a schedule would result in very little time to actually train! In this case, try to taper for the most important events. In addition, concentrate on lower intensity sessions or skills/technique drills the day before the match or event rather than a full-scale workout. The former is likely to cause a lesser degree of glycogen depletion.

How much carbohydrate should be consumed during the rest period?

Your daily intake of carbohydrate during the 48-hour rest period should be as high as 9–10 g/kg. Since your training diet should already be high in carbohydrate, the only change for many females will be the rest from training. If your normal diet contains much less carbohydrate than this, gradually increase the quantity that you are eating during the days leading up to the event.

For some women 9–10 g/kg/day may seem like a huge quantity

Table 1: *Showing the recommended daily carbohydrate intake for females at different body weights in preparation for competition*

Weight	Range of carbohydrate intake (9–10 g/kg/day)
40 kg	360–400 g
50 kg	450–500 g
60 kg	540–600 g
70 kg	630–700 g
80 kg	720–800 g

of carbohydrate. However, such large intakes are necessary to ensure the efficient and complete replenishment of glycogen.

Use the table above to check how much carbohydrate to eat during the rest days before a competition, and refer to chapter 1 for information on which foods you should be eating. Table 1 above should only be used as a guide, since individual circumstances may require you to consume more or less carbohydrate than is recommended. Although it may seem less than scientific, experimentation in training, simulated competitions and minor events is often the most effective way to find out what works best for you.

Put another way, if your event lasts for fewer than 90 minutes, your training diet – which should provide 60% of energy as carbohydrate or 9–10 g/kg/day – coupled with adequate rest will ensure that you have enough fuel on board to last you for the entire event. If, however, your event lasts for longer than 90 minutes, you may want to consider carbohydrate loading (*see* opposite) to boost your carbohydrate intake to up to 70% of your calorie intake or more than 10 g/kg/day.

Menu guides

The following menus are designed to supply a carbohydrate intake of approximately 400 g, 600 g and 800 g. They are ideal for use during the two to three days prior to a major competition. Whilst they meet the requirements for carbohydrate, they are

400 g carbohydrate from:	600 g carbohydrate from:	800 g carbohydrate from:
Breakfast	*Breakfast*	*Breakfast*
Cornflakes (large bowl) with sugar and skimmed milk	2 bananas on 4 slices of toast	Sweetened cereal (large bowl) with skimmed milk
Chopped banana with raisins	1 pint fruit juice	Currant bun (with scraping of butter)
½ pint fruit juice		Handful grapes
		1 pint fruit juice
Snack	*Snack*	*Snack*
1 apple	1 Pop Tart	1 pint flavoured milk (low fat)
		2 scotch pancakes and syrup
Lunch	*Lunch*	*Lunch*
Ham and salad sandwich (2 slices of bread, no butter)	Medium deep pan pizza (ham and pineapple) with salad	1 tin of beans with 4 slices of toast
Low fat yoghurt	Low fat yoghurt	Bowl of jelly and fruit
1 orange	1 pear	Glass of cordial
1 pint cordial	½ pint fruit juice	
Snack	*Snack*	*Snack*
Scone and jam (no butter)	2 crumpets with jam and butter	Bowl of sweetened cereal with skimmed milk
		1 banana

400 g carbohydrate from:	600 g carbohydrate from:	800 g carbohydrate from:
Dinner	*Dinner*	*Dinner*
Large jacket potato (no butter)	Large plate rice (100 g dry weight)	Large portion pasta (100 g dry weight)
Cottage cheese with tuna filling	Small portion chilli con carne (150 g)	Bolognese sauce (150 g)
Large salad	Sweetcorn and peas	Broccoli and carrots
Tin of fruit salad	Yoghurt, banana & dry cereal	Fruit crumble with low fat custard
	$\frac{1}{2}$ pint fruit juice	$\frac{1}{2}$ pint of cordial
	Supper	*Supper*
	1 can low fat rice pudding	2 slices of toast Scraping of butter Honey
ALSO	*ALSO*	*ALSO*
1 litre of isotonic-type sports drink through the day	1 litre of cordial through the day	1 litre of cordial through the day
2000 kcals (8400 kJ)	3400 kcals (14280 kJ)	4000 kcals (166800 kJ)
74% of calories = carbohydrate	66% of calories = carbohydrate	75% of calories = carbohydrate
13% = fat	23% = fat	14% of calories = fat
13% = protein	11% = protein	11% = protein

extremely low in fat and therefore may not necessarily be suitable for everyday use.

In some cases you may discover that you will need to consume more carbohydrate and that your training diet does not meet the recommendations above. If additional carbohydrate is required over and above your everyday intake, follow the guidelines given in table 2.

Beware of increasing the amount of fat that you are eating. It is easy to get carried away so that in an attempt to boost the carbohydrate content of your diet the fat intake creeps up as well! In fact, fat consumption during a taper period should be further reduced to ensure that your calorie intake remains the same. Otherwise you may experience a gain in weight.

This becomes essential during a taper which last longer than a few days. A corresponding decrease in energy intake should be planned to match the reduced work load. Calories should be reduced by eating less fat. At no time should you reduce the carbohydrate content of your diet. Remember, excess dietary fat is very efficiently stored as fat.

There is no need to stuff to the point of discomfort! A successful

Table 2: *A practical guide to boosting the carbohydrate content of your diet in preparation for a competition*

> ♦ Reduce the fat and protein component of the meal and add extra carbohydrate. For example, have an extra potato and less meat, an extra spoonful of rice/pasta and a spoonful less oily/creamy sauce or you might add an extra spoonful of beans and omit the fat from the toast
>
> ♦ Choose a thick-base pizza rather than a thin and crispy one but cut down on the fatty toppings, i.e. more tomato, vegetables, ham, tuna, pineapple and less cheese
>
> ♦ Drink extra juices, squashes or sports drinks with your meals. This adds additional carbohydrate with no extra fat
>
> ♦ Add dried fruit, chopped banana or sugar to breakfast cereal
>
> ♦ Add sugar to hot drinks
>
> ♦ Choose high carbohydrate, low fat snacks such as dried fruit, sweetened popcorn (not buttered), jelly cubes, sugar confectionery, dried breakfast cereal, rusks, bananas

regime will involve eating small to moderate high-carbohydrate, low-fat meals and snacks to meet the recommendations given in table 1.

Remember:

+ to maintain hydration at all times by drinking plenty of fluids
+ to stick to a familiar nutrition programme and avoid any new, untried practices or foods which may negatively affect your performance
+ to think ahead and predict any problems which might occur. Always be prepared to take food with you, particularly if you are staying away from home or travelling abroad.

What about weight-class sports?

Weight-control sports may pose additional problems. Traditional methods of making weight include restriction of food and fluids, use of sweat-suits, saunas, laxatives and diuretics. Clearly such methods will compromise performance due to a combination of reduced glycogen levels and dehydration.

Safe, effective weight loss which does not negatively affect performance can only be achieved by a gradual reduction in fat consumption. This in turn will lead to a reduction in body fat content. This strategy will involve planning to 'make weight' weeks before the start of the competition and not at the last minute as is often the case.

Carbohydrate and fluid intake must be maintained at all times in order to support the training load. A reduction in carbohydrate intake will lead to an inability to train and compete properly as a result of reduced glycogen stores. Similarly, dehydration can reduce exercise capacity and adversely affect performance.

A major problem with increasing the carbohydrate content of the diet in the week prior to the event is that the extra carbohydrate, stored with water as glycogen, causes you to weigh heavier. Whilst this extra glycogen is an advantage for most females, it can be a disadvantage in weight-dominated sports where the category is often reached by the narrowest of margins.

This highlights the importance of forward planning so that

weight is made in advance and the female is able to maintain a high-carbohydrate diet accompanied by plenty of fluids. The advantage of such preparation is obvious and any females who follow this strategy will be at a huge advantage over their competitors.

What is carbohydrate loading?

Carbohydrate loading is the term used to describe the elevation above normal levels of muscle glycogen levels. It is sometimes referred to as *supercompensation*.

The traditional or 'classical' regime involves completing an exhausting training session followed by a low-carbohydrate, high-protein and high-fat diet. This depletion phase is maintained for three to four days in order to increase the levels of the enzyme responsible for storing glycogen in the muscle. If the muscle is then 'crammed' with plenty of carbohydrate, i.e. the individual switches to an extremely high carbohydrate diet, then additional glycogen is stored.

In practice such a regime is unpleasant to follow. Problems frequently occur during the depletion phase with athletes experiencing fatigue and gastro-intestinal upsets from the high protein/ fat diet. They may also suffer mood swings and irritability.

Despite this, many females ranging from sprinters to ultra-distance participants confess to having tried carbohydrate loading.

Is it possible to carbohydrate load without a depletion phase?

The simple answer is yes. In the light of the problems associated with such a regime, American researchers have developed a modified glycogen loading programme which is as effective as the classical method and can increase muscle glycogen stores to up to 20–40% above normal.

The modified programme is similar to the normal preparation for competition except that the taper period is extended and slightly more carbohydrate is consumed.

On days seven to four prior to the event, a normal mixed diet should be eaten. This will typically contain less carbohydrate than you are used to eating (approximately 50% of energy). Training should be moderately hard (1–2 hrs/day). Three days before the start, training should be reduced to no more than 60 minutes of low intensity work accompanied by a carbohydrate intake of *at least* 9–10 g/day (or up to 70% of energy).

Since this scheme will almost certainly require you to consume more carbohydrate than normal, follow the guidelines given in table 2 (page 153) for some ideas. A word of caution, however: don't get carried away and end up fat-loading as well! Focus your food choices on high-carbohydrate, low fat meals and snacks. Fluid intake should remain high at all times.

Carbohydrate loading is mainly relevant in events which involve over 90 minutes of continuous, high-intensity activity which stress the same muscle groups. Such exercise will challenge the female's normal fuel stores. There is, however, a small amount of evidence which indicates that carbohydrate loading may also improve performance during maximal exercise which only lasts several minutes.

If you have experienced a drop in pace or a reduction in performance in conjunction with feelings of muscle glycogen depletion towards the end of an event then you may benefit from this procedure. Always experiment in a minor competition or under simulated event conditions to ensure that it works for you. Never try this for the first time in preparation for an important competition.

What should be eaten for the pre-competition meal?

Traditionally it was believed that a high-protein meal would set you up for the day's events. It is still common to hear reports of footballers tucking into steak, eggs and chips or munching their way through steak-and-kidney pies prior to a match! This type of meal offers little in the way of carbohydrate and is less than ideal for the nutrition-conscious competitor.

The aims of the pre-event meal are to top up glycogen stores (muscle glycogen stores should already be full if you have organised your preparation well, but liver glycogen stores may need replenishing), to maintain hydration, to stave off hunger and to give the competitor a psychological boost.

Foods ingested during this period should be high in carbohydrate and low in fat since high fat foods are digested more slowly. They should also be low in fibre and bulk. This is particularly important for females who are prone to pre-event nerves, diarrhoea or 'the trots'. Always choose foods which are well tolerated and which have a high to moderate glycaemic index (*see* page 8) to ensure rapid digestion and absorption.

Research suggests that performance can be improved when a carbohydrate-rich meal is consumed three to four hours before prolonged exercise. In one particular study, cyclists improved their power output by 22% when they consumed 200 g of carbohydrate from bread, cereals and fruit four hours prior to exercising, as well as a chocolate bar (43 g sucrose) five minutes before exercise. This is because a relatively large pre-exercise meal appears to increase performance by maintaining a high use of carbohydrate later on in endurance exercise.

Lesser amounts of carbohydrate (i.e. 50–150 g) have not produced the same responses.

Practically, however, 200 g of carbohydrate can be bulky to consume! Some females may not be able to tolerate this quantity of carbohydrate even if some of it is in fluid form.

The essential thing is that the meal should not cause any discomfort or feelings of bloatedness. As a result, the timing of the meal and quantity of food eaten will vary from individual to individual despite the fact that studies recommend ingesting 200–300 g of carbohydrate during the four hours prior to exercise.

The key is to find out what works for you and stick to it. As a general rule, if a large meal is consumed then leave three or four hours for it to digest. If you consume a pre-event snack then leave between one and two hours. If you are involved in a sport which requires a weigh-in then you will probably leave your pre-event meal until afterwards.

Some ideas for pre-event meals and snacks are listed in table 3. These should always be accompanied by some fluid.

If solid foods cannot be tolerated during this time then use liquid meals such as carbohydrate supplements (for example Isostar Long Energy, Maxim, High 5, PSP22, Ultra-Fuel) or sports drinks (for example Gatorade, Isostar, Lucozade Sport), high carbohydrate baby foods, or rusks with low-fat milk or jelly.

It is vital to continue to drink up to the start of your first event. Carry a drinks bottle with you at all times and choose sports drinks, diluted juices, cordial or water.

Table 3: *Pre-event meals and snacks*

Breakfast cereal and low fat milk
Toast (scraping of fat) with honey/jam
Banana or jam sandwiches
Muffins/crumpets with jam/honey
Pancakes and syrup
Beans on toast
Pasta with tomato-based sauce
Jacket potato with low fat filling
Canned fruit
Low fat rice pudding
Currant buns/scones with jam
Rusks and low fat milk

Remember: choose white bread and lower fibre cereals, and avoid high-fibre foods such as beans if you suffer from any intestinal or bowel problems unless you are sure that you can tolerate them

If you find that you become hungry prior to the start, then have a small, carbohydrate-rich snack. Ignoring hunger pangs will cause you to focus on your stomach rather than the competition – so have something to eat!

Should sugary products be consumed within one hour of an event?

Many females believe that sugar consumption should be avoided prior to exercising. The belief arises from suggestions that such a practice may upset blood sugar levels and suppress the metabolism of fatty acids, ultimately causing glycogen to be used more quickly than normal.

These recommendations appear to arise from one or two studies – conducted as long ago as 1977 – which reported a negative effect of ingesting sugar just prior to performance. Subsequent studies have failed to reproduce these results. Some have demonstrated no effect of sugar intake on performance, but interestingly, more recent work has suggested that sugar ingestion may have an ergogenic effect by actually enhancing performance. The suggested mechanisms for this improvement in performance in endurance events is that the sugar provides extra carbohydrate either to support high rates of carbohydrate oxidation or to maintain blood sugar levels later on in exercise. In any case, there is substantial evidence to show that even if blood sugar levels are disturbed, metabolism reverts back to its normal pattern once exercise has started, with no adverse effect on performance.

Therefore recent reports lead us to conclude that there is little support for the idea that sugar ingestion prior to performance actually impairs performance. Indeed, there is growing evidence to suggest that this may be a useful practice in events where glycogen depletion is a problem.

A recent study by a group of Spanish researchers has indicated that feeding a glucose drink (75 g) to runners 30 minutes prior to a run of high intensity and intermediate duration can significantly improve the time to exhaustion compared with drinking plain water or fructose. This suggests that the advantages of sugar feeding prior to performance may not be limited to prolonged events.

Anyone who believes that they may benefit from a small, sugar-rich snack (approximately 50 g) prior to exercise should experiment in training or minor competitions first. Anecdotal evidence suggests that exercisers tolerate the carbohydrate better in the form of fluid confectionery (for example chocolate, turkish delight, jelly babies, jelly beans or energy bars).

What about fluid intake?

Dehydration will impair exercise capacity and can cause serious risks to health. Dehydration may impair performance when as little as 2% of body weight is lost through sweating (i.e. 1.2 kg for a 60 kg female). It is essential that hydration is maintained at all times over a competition, even if you are involved in an activity which requires you to 'make weight'.

Weight and urine checks provide practical ways to monitor your fluid status. A weight reduction of 1 kg over a session is the equivalent of 1 litre of sweat lost. A simple 'before' and 'after' weight check can help a female to determine her fluid requirements. In addition, frequent visits to the toilet and the production of copious quantities of pale-coloured urine indicates adequate hydration. In contrast, a lesser quantity of dark-coloured, smelly urine indicates dehydration.

During short, high-intensity events such as sprinting, middle-distance track events, competitive swimming events, judo bouts and other exercise periods lasting up to 30 minutes it is not usually necessary, nor is it often possible, to consume fluid during the event. This is presuming that the female competitor is well hydrated prior to the start and continues to compensate for fluid losses between bouts of exercise. However, it is difficult to identify a cut-off point beyond which fluid consumption becomes essential, since many factors will influence the individual's requirements.

If exercise is of a longer duration, fluid replacement during exercise is usually necessary since sweat losses can be high and there is a real risk of dehydration if fluid is not consumed.

Opportunities to take fluid on board should be organised during longer events. Drinks breaks should be scheduled and competitors should make use of any available opportunity to consume some fluid. This is particularly important during events where the rules dictate the opportunity to drink – for example, in many team games.

The amount of fluid that is drunk will depend on a number of factors. During prolonged activity where large sweat losses are predicted, it is recommended that fluid is ingested before, during and after exercise at regular intervals. It is recommended to start the event with the maximum quantity of fluid tolerable in your stomach. This should be topped up during the activity.

A fluid intake of 150–250 ml per 15 minutes is often recommended, although there are clear problems associated with making such hard and fast rules. The key is to practise drinking and to offset weight losses of more than 1% of your total body weight.

What drinks are recommended?

A dilute carbohydrate–electrolyte drink will deliver water faster to the tissues than plain water. This is because small amounts of glucose and sodium stimulate the uptake of water in the intestine. Hence the reason why some sports drinks (such as Isostar and Gatorade) are formulated to contain both these ingredients.

Consumption of a well-formulated sports drink during prolonged, high-intensity exercise (1–3 hours continuous) when sweat losses are high is essential to ensure that fluid needs are met.

In shorter events, where sweat losses are not significant, a number of drinks are suitable such as water, diluted fruit juice or fruit cordial. It is unlikely that fluid or fuel deficits will be serious in shorter events. However, it is prudent to err on the side of caution and to take fluid on board just in case.

During the event – food or fluid?

Sports drinks have the added advantage of containing a substantial quantity of carbohydrate (between 50–80 g/litre). As a result they can meet the dual requirements for energy and fluid during exercise.

Carbohydrate feedings during an event appear to be of little benefit in activities that are not limited by carbohydrate availability. Such events include sprint swimming and running, baseball, cricket and figure skating.

However, carbohydrate feeding during prolonged exercise has been shown to delay fatigue by preventing hypoglycaemia and maintaining high rates of glucose use. The effects of such feedings are clear in cyclists but less obvious in running events. Since the amount of carbohydrate available later in exercise will influence performance, it seems reasonable to suggest that it may be of benefit to consume carbohydrate in events of a continuous nature which last longer than 60 minutes.

Recent research has also indicated that a carbohydrate drink consumed during prolonged exercise may help to maintain white-cell functioning; this might in turn reduce the risk of becoming ill once the exercise is over. Further research is required to substantiate this.

If glycogen stores are reduced prior to the start of the exercise (a situation which is common amongst participants), then carbohydrate supplementation will have a more immediate effect.

During extreme activities such as road races, triathlon and ultra-distance running, sailing and distance canoeing, females may also desire food. This can contribute to an increased carbohydrate intake. High glycaemic index foods should be selected and be accompanied by fluid. Common choices include:

♦ energy bars, confectionery and muesli bars
♦ raisins and bananas
♦ sugar confectionery

+ jelly cubes
+ sandwiches
+ Pop Tarts
+ tinned fruit.

Carbohydrate feedings are also of benefit in high-intensity, intermittent activities such as football, hockey and tennis. Such exercises are glycogen depleting, so the benefits may be due to the glycogen sparing effects of the feedings.

How much carbohydrate should be consumed during exercise?

Research suggests that sufficient carbohydrate should be consumed to supply approximately 1 g/minute.

Many of the studies in this area have used protocols which involved feeding subjects between 30–60 g carbohydrate per hour to produce an ergogenic effect. Researchers from The University of Maastrict in The Netherlands showed that the ingestion of 50 g of carbohydrate at the start of exercise followed by 12–13 g each 15 minutes led to near maximal rates of oxidation of these carbohydrate supplements during a 2-hour cycle exercise.

The 30–60 g range should only be used as a guidance which should be adapted more specifically to the individual's circumstances. Trial and error and a bit of logic will help to determine exactly how much carbohydrate is needed.

One litre of an isotonic type of sports drink will supply approximately 70 g carbohydrate. Therefore the regular consumption of a sports drink, starting early in exercise, provides a convenient method of meeting both fluid and carbohydrate needs.

What about all-day events?

Competitions often last all day, and may continue for several days. In such tournament situations women may be competing several times each day with variable amounts of rest in-between bouts of exercise. The question always arises as to what to eat and drink between sessions.

Food choices will be influenced by several factors, including the length of time between events, food availability and individual preferences. However, women should use these breaks to top up glycogen stores and replenish fluid levels.

As a general rule, when there is less than one hour between events it is wise to stick to sports drinks and other soft drinks. Food intake may be a problem due to the limited time for digestion and absorption and the possibility of gastric discomfort. Having said this, some competitors may choose to eat a light carbohydrate snack at this time.

If there are 2–4 hours between events, a light, carbohydrate-rich meal will help to begin to restore glycogen to its pre-exercise levels.

Use the table below to identify ideas for snacks and meals.

Table 4: Guidelines for eating at all-day events

Less than one hour	2–4 hours
Sports drinks (e.g. Isostar, Gatorade, Lucozade Sport) Carbohydrate supplements (e.g. GatorLode, Maxim, High 5, PSP22, UltraFuel) Soft drinks (diluted fruit juice and cordial) *Possibly*: Bananas and raisins Energy bars Confectionery Jelly cubes Sugar confectionery (e.g. jelly babies, jelly beans, Licorice Allsorts) Plain biscuits Rice cakes	Sandwiches/rolls/pitta Currant buns/tea-cakes Bagels/muffins/crumpets Scones/scotch pancakes Toast/toasted sandwiches Cereal/rusks Pop Tarts Popcorn Canned fruit or dried fruit Low fat rice pudding Pasta and tomato sauce Jacket potato Rice and low fat sauce
Remember: Keep drinking at all times! Keep the fat content of the meal low! Do not stuff! Eat small amounts and often.	

Is there a special post-competition strategy?

Once the competition has completely finished, then it is time to celebrate and to give yourself a well-deserved rest. If, however, you are competing the following day or within the next few days your post-event food intake is crucial.

Muscle glycogen resynthesis is faster than normal immediately after exercise. Women should aim to take some carbohydrate on board (approximately 1 g/kg) as soon after exercise as is practical. This will probably be in the form of fluid or a carbohydrate-rich snack.

This should be followed by a carbohydrate-rich meal consumed approximately 2 hours later. Some research has shown that muscle glycogen resynthesis may be near optimal when at least 50 g of carbohydrate is consumed at 2-hour intervals.

The latest studies from Ohio State University have proposed a strategy which may increase the rate of glycogen storage by up to 20% over and above the 50 g/2 hours regime outlined above. The study involved exhaustive exercise which severely reduced the subject's muscle glycogen levels. Following each workout, subjects consumed carbohydrate every 15 minutes for 4 hours! This pattern of eating is sometimes called 'grazing'. The amount of carbohydrate consumed was enormous – almost 3 g/lb or 6 g/kg of body weight (more than many people consume in a day and over half the daily recommendation for individuals in heavy training)! This was then sub-divided into 16 equal doses over the 4-hour period. This meant that the athletes were ingesting about 30 g of carbohydrate every 15 minutes! Imagine eating 2 bananas every 15 minutes for 4 hours after exercise, or consuming 500 ml of sports drink in the same way!

Muscle biopsies revealed that 20% more glycogen was stored than when 50 g of carbohydrate is consumed every 2 hours.

It is possible that this 15-minute strategy is so effective because it ensures high blood glucose and insulin levels over a 4-hour period, therefore enhancing glycogen storage.

Before you rush out to try this plan it must be stressed that the subjects had participated in exhaustive exercise prior to the 'loading' programme. It is likely that such a scheme will only be relevant for women who are involved in activities which are severely glycogen depleting.

It may be a useful strategy to employ during periods of intensive training or if you are competing more than once a day. As with all these programmes, it may not be suitable for everyone and must be tried and tested in training first. From a practical viewpoint it may be impossible for a person to consume that amount (over half your daily requirement) of carbohydrate in 4 hours. Such schemes should be carefully planned with the help of a qualified sports nutritionist.

A modified version of this plan, and one which would be easier to achieve from a practical point of view, involves consuming the recommended post-event carbohydrate-rich snack, then continuing to consume fluid (containing some carbohydrate) until a meal is consumed. In this way a continuous stream of carbohydrate is supplied to the muscles.

SUMMARY

+ Taper training and maintain a high-carbohydrate diet (9–10 g/kg) in the days prior to a competition to ensure maximal storage of glycogen.
+ Women involved in events where carbohydrate availability is a limiting factor may benefit from carbohydrate loading.
+ Drink plenty of fluids to offset dehydration.
+ Avoid practices which cause dehydration or glycogen depletion to make a weight category.
+ Ensure that pre-event meals and snacks are carbohydrate-rich, low in fat, fibre and bulk.
+ Drink before, during (if relevant) and after the event.
+ Top up glycogen stores with suitable high-carbohydrate foods and drinks during (where necessary) the event and between events.
+ Ensure that you follow an adequate refuelling and rehydration plan if competing on subsequent days.

PRACTICAL POINTS

+ Never try anything new during the period before an event. Stick to a tried and tested regime.
+ Try out new ideas and plans in training or at less important events.
+ Plan ahead and always pack suitable snacks and drinks in your kit bag.
+ If you have any doubts about your preparation, then consult a qualified sports nutritionist.

References

F. Brouns, *Nutritional Needs of Athletes* (John Wiley & Sons, Chichester, 1993)

D.L. Costill, M. Hargreaves, *Carbohydrate Nutrition and Fatigue* (Sports Medicine, 13, 86–92, 1992)

J. Fallowfield, C. Williams, *Carbohydrate Intake and Recovery from Prolonged Exercise* (International Journal of Sports Nutrition, 3, 150–164, 1993)

Food Nutrition and Sports Performance – Proceedings of an International Scientific Consensus (Journal of Sports Sciences, 9, Special Issue, Summer 1991)

Foods, Nutrition and Soccer Performance – Proceedings of an International Scientific Consensus (Journal of Sports Sciences, 12, Special Issue, Summer 1994)

P.D. Neufer et al., *Improvements in Exercise Performance: Effects of Carbohydrate Feedings and Diet* (Journal of Applied Physiology, 63, 983–8, 1987)

J.G. Seifert et al., *Glycaemic and Insulinemic Response to Preexercise Carbohydrate Feedings* (International Journal of Sport Nutrition, 4, 1, March 1994)

J.L. Ventura et al., *Effect of Prior Ingestion of Glucose or Fructose on the Performance of Exercise of Intermediate Duration* (European Journal of Applied Physiology, 68, 345–349, 1994)

A.J.M. Wagenmakers et al., *Oxidation Rates of Orally Ingested Carbohydrates During Prolonged Exercise* (Journal of Applied Physiology, 75 (6), 2774–80, December 1994)

MAKING WEIGHT

Jane Griffin

Jane Griffin qualified from London University with a degree in Nutrition and a Postgraduate Diploma in Dietetics. After working for several years in industry for a variety of food and pharmaceutical companies she set up her own nutritional and dietetic consultancy 12 years ago. She has specialised in spreading the 'healthy eating' message via media work with women's magazines, radio and television. Over the last eight years she has also become more and more involved in the area of sports nutrition. She is the Consultant Nutritionist to the British Olympic Association and travelled with the Great Britain team to the Barcelona Olympic Games in 1992. Jane has written for *Running* magazine and *Squash Player* for several years, as well as for *Athletics Weekly*, *Martial Arts Today* and *Performance Cyclist*. She now writes for *Karate World* and the *Bike Mag*.

Most female athletes find that they perform best at a particular body weight or at least within a narrow range of body weights. For some athletes, however, their sport dictates that they *must* compete at a particular weight – one which is seldom their natural one. As a result, they have to lose weight.

This is usually done by *making weight*, so called because an athlete must weigh a certain amount in order to 'make' a weight class prior to competition. Such sports include martial arts, weight-lifting, wrestling and lightweight rowing. Other athletes such as body-builders, dancers and figure-skaters may need to make weight to improve appearance, while gymnasts and jockeys may lose weight close to competing by dehydration in the hope of increasing stamina and power relative to body weight.

Weight classes are determined by the particular sport's governing body. In the case of lightweight rowing, women row at a maximum body weight of 59 kg with an average crew weight of 57 kg. In other sports, weight classes are intended to eliminate injuries which could arise if competitors were ill-matched physically, or to allow athletes of all sizes to compete on an equal basis. Unfortunately, it does not necessarily work like that. Many athletes lose weight to qualify for a lower weight class in the belief that they will have the advantage of size, strength, power and leverage over their opponent. In other words, they seek to compete at a weight where the power to weight ratio is optimal, where muscle mass is maximised and body fat minimised to gain competitive advantage.

How is weight made?

Some athletes keep their body weight continually low by following a strict diet all the year round. Others lose weight during the season and gain it off-season, and still others lose and gain weight repeatedly throughout the season (and from season to season). A variety of rapid weight loss methods are used, particularly by this latter group.

+ *Food restriction* – severe reduction in total energy (or calorie) intake
+ *Starvation* – complete avoidance of food for one or more days before weigh-in
+ *Fluid restriction* – rationing or complete avoidance of fluid intake one or more days before weigh-in
+ *Heat exposure* – use of saunas, steam rooms and hot showers to encourage weight loss by dehydration through sweating
+ *Strenuous exercise* – long, hard training sessions to encourage weight loss by dehydration through sweating. Sweat rate is

often increased by wearing extra clothing, for example track suits, woollen hats and scarves or sweatsuits during the session

♦ *Diuretics* – to stimulate the kidneys to produce more urine, increase fluid losses and therefore increase weight loss

♦ *Vomiting and laxatives* – to ensure that the stomach is empty and that all waste products are removed, thus making the body as 'light' as possible

What are the problems of making weight?

It can be seen that the basic principles of making weight are either to cut back food intake so severely that the body has to call on its own stores to supply the energy deficit, or to reduce the body's total water content by dehydration or restriction of fluid intake. The outcome of such practices can affect health and performance depending on the severity of the method used and how frequently the athlete has to make weight.

Table 1: Example of poor glycogen refuelling on a low-calorie diet

> ♦ A female judokas has already managed to get her weight down from 60 kg to 58 kg but wishes to compete in the lightweight category (up to 56 kg).
>
> ♦ Her present daily calorie intake is 1500 kcals and her carbohydrate intake is 225 g (60% of total energy intake).
>
> ♦ On a weight basis her carbohydrate intake works out at 3.9 g per kg body weight per day. This amount of carbohydrate would not be enough to replenish muscle glycogen stores on a daily basis.
>
> ♦ She drops her intake to 1000 kcals per day in an attempt to get her weight down to 56 kg. If she keeps to a carbohydrate intake of 60% of total energy, this will only provide 2.6 g per kg body weight per day.
>
> ♦ If she attempts to train hard in order to keep up the weight loss, she could well end up at the competition 'dead at the weight'.

What are the problems with a restricted food intake?

Although the overall aim is to reduce energy or calorie intake, the intake of essential nutrients such as vitamins, minerals, carbohydrate and protein may also be impaired.

- *Carbohydrate* – strict dieting or starvation causes a fall in muscle and liver glycogen levels. This can lead to fatigue and poor performance, particularly in endurance events such as rowing. In other sports the effect may be cumulative during a competition and become apparent as an athlete advances through the rounds. Complete replenishment of severely depleted muscle glycogen stores can take up to 48 hours.
- *Protein* – in a similar way, protein intake may be inadequate for athletic performance. Recent research suggests that strength or speed athletes should consume about 1.2–1.7 g protein per kg body weight per day and endurance athletes about 1.2–1.4 g per kg body weight per day. (The requirement for non-athletic adults is 0.75 g per kg body weight per day.) A restricted energy intake can lead to negative nitrogen balance at protein intakes that promote positive nitrogen balance when energy intake is adequate. Repeated attempts to make weight throughout a season could compromise protein metabolism and thus affect performance.
- *Micronutrients* – intake of minerals and vitamins may be less than optimal, though actual signs of deficiency may not be seen. Iron and calcium intakes are often low in female athletes because of poor food choices, avoidance of iron- and calcium-rich foods and poor eating habits (irregular meals and heavy reliance on snacking). Restricting food intake even more in order to make weight can only exacerbate the situation.

What are the problems with dehydration?

A weight loss of as little as 2% of body weight can impair performance. Body water is found predominantly in lean tissue – muscles, blood and vital organs – but not in body fat tissue. Dehydration by any method leads to a fall in plasma volume which in turn can lead to a fall in cardiac output, a rise in heart rate and a fall in blood pressure. It can also contribute to a drop in blood flow to the kidneys, skin and muscles. As the body becomes more dehydrated, the ability to produce sweat falls off and the temperature regulation mechanism is compromised. Prolonged exercise or heat exposure in a dehydrated state can ultimately lead to heat exhaustion or heat stroke.

Diuretics cause a greater loss of fluid from the circulation than any other method of dehydration. They also give rise to losses of sodium and chloride from the blood and potassium and magnesium from muscle cells. Losses of minerals and water together can increase the risk of muscle cramps and spasms. The use of diuretics is not recommended and indeed the IOC has added diuretics to the list of drugs banned for use by athletes in Olympic competition. Many governing bodies have also banned them.

Dehydration does not affect muscle glycogen stores unless the dehydration has been achieved by undergoing strenuous exercise to increase sweat losses. However, if dehydration is accompanied by restricted food intake, total body water content and muscle glycogen stores will both be depleted.

What effects can rapid weight loss have on performance?

The effects of rapid weight loss on aerobic performance are adverse and profound. There is however conflicting evidence from studies on the effects, particularly of dehydration, of making weight on 'high-power' performance. Dehydration does not appear to adversely affect such performance lasting less than 30 seconds. However, the ability to sustain near maximal efforts for more than 30 seconds may be reduced.

Finally, rapid weight loss can cause mood changes that have a negative influence on performance; the general symptoms associated with starvation – tiredness, nausea and dizziness – can be very detrimental.

Is there a health hazard to yo-yo dieting?

Yo-yo dieting is the term used to describe repeated cycles of weight loss and weight gain. A very restricted calorie diet is usually followed, producing an initial weight loss. However, the diet is often difficult to follow and certainly hard to maintain, with the result that when it is finally abandoned the weight returns (often

171

with more besides). The cycle is then repeated, but each time the dieter finds it harder and harder to maintain the weight loss.

Until recently, the accepted explanation for this was that the metabolic rate falls during the dieting period as the body adapts to a state of semi-starvation and learns to survive on fewer calories. This lower metabolic rate was thought to be maintained after dieting stopped so that, in effect, less calories were needed to maintain weight. A return to the pre-dieting calorie intake would therefore result in further weight increases.

Such a theory is now being questioned. Metabolism is certainly suppressed each time one diets, but – contrary to popular belief – research carried out at the Medical Research Council's Dunn Nutrition Unit in Cambridge shows that the metabolic rate bounces back up again when the diet is stopped. At the Dunn, they showed that after three yo-yo cycles the metabolic rate was exactly the same as when the group of dieters started – *and* they were 12 lb lighter. Regular dieting does not therefore permanently damage your metabolism.

One explanation for the 'apparent' resistance to progressive attempts to lose weight is the emotional strain and sheer frustration of yo-yo dieting. The women in the Cambridge study admitted that they were fed up with the diet by the time the third dieting phase came and they certainly cheated more during the last diet cycle. Yo-yo dieting seems to be more of a problem if a rapid weight loss method such as a very restricted calorie diet is used.

There is some concern that in the long term, weight cycling may lead to certain health risks such as an increase in coronary heart disease and high blood pressure or hypertension.

How can you make weight safely?

There are three areas to be considered when planning a programme to make weight. First, body weight should be controlled in the off-season so that the amount of weight that has to be lost during the training phase and run-up to competition can be achieved without severe calorie restrictions or anything more than a minimal weight loss by dehydration. Second, a realistic competition weight should be agreed. Third, weight loss should

Table 2: *Typical example of weight bands for a lightweight female rower*

Competition weight	57 kg
Training weight	57–60 kg
Living weight	60–62 kg

be gradual and achieved by using sound nutritional practices to ensure an increase in the ratio of lean body mass to body fat.

How can I control my off-season weight?

Each athlete has a 'living' weight band, a 'training' weight band and a realistic competition weight. These weight bands differ for individual athletes.

Athletes who have to control their weight during the competition season like to 'live normally' during the time between the end of the season and the start of the new season's training programme. During this time they eat and drink without restrictions, snack and eat meals and enjoy the foods they denied themselves all season. The more weight they put on during this time, the more weight will have to be lost once training begins. Many athletes do not bother to weigh themselves at all during this time and so have no way of checking on weight gain. By setting an upper limit to the living weight band, and by monitoring weight by weekly weighings, a certain amount of damage limitation can be achieved.

How can I decide on a competition weight?

The ideal way to determine your weight category for a new season is to enlist the help of a qualified sports dietitian or nutritionist. They will be able to estimate your minimal weight. This is done by measuring your body fat and then calculating how much fat you can afford to lose without affecting health or performance. The actual amount of weight you can afford to lose is then calculated by subtracting the minimal weight from your present weight. Such a calculation should help you to determine your realistic weight category. As a general guide, if you always have to lose 5 kg (11 lb) or more to make weight, you should reconsider the weight category you are competing in.

How should the weight loss be achieved?

A well-planned dietary strategy should enable you to lose slowly and steadily while still maintaining your training programme. You should aim for a maximum weekly weight loss of 0.5– 1.0 kg (1–2 lb). Ideally, you should reach your competition weight between three and five days before you have to weigh in. Certainly you should be very close to weight two or three days prior to the competition, with nothing left to do but a little fine tuning.

To achieve a weight loss of 0.5 kg per week there has to be a weekly deficit of 3500 kcals. Daily calorie deficits therefore need to be 500–1000 kcals. The overall intake should never fall below 1200 kcals per day, and during more intensive phases of your training programme you will need to increase to 1500 or even 1800 kcals per day if you are going to refuel effectively after each training session. Be guided by your weekly weight loss and by how your training is going as to whether you are achieving the right intake. Too rapid a weight loss, and you will need to increase your intake; no weight loss over two weeks, and you will need to cut back more.

The carbohydrate intake should be as high as possible to promote glycogen synthesis. A high proportion of starchy carbo-hydrate foods should be included to add bulk to the diet. Fat content needs to be reduced to a maximum of 25% of total energy, and protein needs to be maintained at a minimum of 15% of total energy. It is important to select foods which are *nutrient dense*, i.e. low in calories but high in nutritional value, if the requirements of vitamins and minerals are to be met.

So what should you eat?

The emphasis of your diet should be on bread, pasta, rice, pota-toes (jacket or boiled), breakfast cereals (preferably fortified with iron), pulses (peas, beans, lentils), fruits and fruit juices and vegetables. You should also include low fat dairy foods such as skimmed or semi skimmed milk, diet yoghurts and low fat cheeses (cottage cheese, low fat soft cheese) to ensure an adequate intake of calcium. If you eat meat, include some lean red meat to help maintain your iron intake, but also include chicken (no skin) and fish. Vegetarians should include pulses, quorn, tofu and eggs to ensure a good intake of protein. Cheese is a good source of protein but most varieties also have high fat contents. To boost iron intake, you should try to have a bowl of iron-fortified breakfast cereal with low-fat milk and a glass of orange juice. The vitamin C in the juice helps the body to absorb the iron in the cereal which is otherwise not very well absorbed. Include a variety of vegetables, particularly broccoli, spinach, green peppers, tomatoes and carrots as well as lots of fruit. Fruit and vegetables tend to be low in calories yet provide a range of vitamins in reasonable amounts.

As the intake of vitamins will probably decrease with decreasing calorie intake, it is a good idea to take a multivitamin supplement with iron on a daily basis if only as an insurance policy. However, it is important that you choose the correct type. You need to buy a supplement which gives you 100% of the RDA (Recommended Daily Amount) and no more. There is no benefit from taking megadoses of vitamins.

▲
PRACTICAL POINTS
▼

+ If you still need to lose weight in the last 7–10 days, reduce your energy intake slightly (especially if you are tapering down). However, you need to maintain your intake of carbohydrates so be even stricter with the fats: no fat on bread, skimmed milk only.
+ Reduce your salt intake by not adding salt at the table or in cooking and by avoiding high salt foods (many of which are high in fat anyway).
+ Have a *low fibre* diet for the last 24 hours – switch to white bread, low fibre breakfast cereals, etc.
+ Post weigh-in, start rehydrating as soon as possible if you have had to do any last minute dehydrating. How effective this will be will depend on the amount of body weight lost through dehydration and the time you have between weighing-in and competing.
+ What to drink? Having plain water makes you feel less thirsty and less inclined to drink; it also stimulates urine production. Both these factors will delay the rehydration process. A drink

containing some electrolytes (particularly sodium), some carbohydrate and of course water will help you to rehydrate efficiently. Isotonic sports drinks such as Isostar and Lucozade
Sports are suitable.

Case study – a lightweight female rower

♦ JB started rowing when she was 18. She was a skinny girl
and not worried about weight at all. Two years later she
became vegetarian and much more aware of what she was
eating. Four years later JB had her first year rowing lightweight. It was the first time in the squad and training was
hard. The weight dropped off easily and she came down
from 60 kg to 57 kg. In fact, she had to eat lots to hold her
weight at 57 kg. During the winter her weight increased to
62 kg (2 kg more than she had ever been before). The next
season JB was asked to drop down to 56 kg. She cut down
the amount of food she was eating, cut out fat and stopped
drinking alcohol. She made weight by diet alone – no
sweating – and managed to keep this weight throughout
the racing season. After a successful World Championship
her weight went up to 65 kg in the winter as she enjoyed a
'normal life'. Then the dieting season started again and JB
had to get down to 56 kg though at the last minute she was
allowed to go to 57 kg. However this time she had to sweat
in order to get to 57 kg.

♦ For the Worlds, JB did have to go down to 56 kg – by calorie
counting, cutting back on carbohydrates and eating lots of
vegetables and pre-packed meals of known calorie content.
JB was now taking 15–20 laxatives a day, doing sweat
paddles and even contemplating cutting her hair off to
help her get to weight. She felt weak and shaky at the
Worlds and did not do well.

♦ The next winter her weight went up to 69 kg and by Easter
it was still at 67 kg. JB's diet was no more than 1200 kcals
and diet cokes figured very strongly as a way of filling up
on no calories. Her weight came down to 63 kg and then
stabilised. Now followed the rhubarb diet (the food with
the lowest calorific value) and more laxatives.

♦ At this stage JB enlisted the help of a sports dietitian who immediately put her on a 1500 kcal diet with a high carbohydrate content and changed her eating habits to maximise refuelling post-training. JB made 59 kg at the Worlds without the use of laxatives or sweating, and she and the rest of the crew came back with the silver medal.

11

EATING PLANS AND SNACKS

Anita Bean and Peggy Wellington

Eating plans

The following plans have been carefully formulated to help you balance and regulate your daily nutritional intake.

Table 1: Sample eating plan providing approx. 2000 calories

Breakfast:	50 g (2 oz) wholegrain breakfast cereal 150 ml (¼ pint) skimmed/semi skimmed milk 1 banana
Snack:	1 apple 1 low fat yoghurt
Lunch:	225 g (8 oz) baked potato 1 tsp (5 ml) low fat spread 100 g (4 oz) tuna mixed with 1 tbsp (15 ml) fromage frais *or* 100 g (4 oz) cottage cheese 1 carton (100 g) low calorie fromage frais 1 orange
Snack:	1 English muffin with low fat spread
Dinner:	200 g (7 oz) chicken leg, grilled and skinned *or* cooked beans Tomato salad with herbs Green salad with 1 tbsp (15 ml) olive oil/vinegar dressing 75 g (3 oz) rice (uncooked weight) 175 g (6 oz) fruit salad **Nutritional information:** **Energy: 1950 kcal; carbohydrate: 318 g (62% of kcal);** **fat: 38 g (18% of kcal); protein: 103 g (20% of kcal)**

Table 2: Sample eating plan providing approx. 2500 calories

Breakfast:	75 g (3 oz) wholegrain breakfast cereal 150 ml (¼ pint) skimmed/semi skimmed milk 1 glass (150 ml/¼ pint) fruit juice 1 slice toast with low fat spread and honey or jam
Snack:	1 mini pitta filled with 50 g (2 oz) cottage cheese 100 g (4 oz) grapes/plums/apricots
Lunch:	1 large wholemeal bap with low fat spread Egg salad filling (1 egg with salad) *or* 75 g (3 oz) chicken and salad 1 low fat yoghurt 1 banana
Snack:	1 fruit scone with jam or fruit spread
Dinner:	100 g (4 oz) pasta (uncooked weight) 100 g (4 oz) Neopolitan sauce mixed with 75 g (3 oz) lean ham/mince/cooked lentils 225 g (8 oz) vegetables or salad 225 g (8 oz) rice pudding 100 g (4 oz) fruit (e.g. apricots, pineapple)
Snack:	3 wholemeal crackers 25 g (1 oz) hard cheese
	Nutritional information: **Energy: 2540 kcal; carbohydrate: 433 g (64% of kcal);** **fat: 56 g (20% of kcal); protein: 103 g (16% of kcal)**

Table 3: Sample eating plan providing approx. 3000 calories

Breakfast:	75 g (3 oz) wholegrain breakfast cereal 300 ml ($\frac{1}{2}$ pint) skimmed/semi skimmed milk 1 glass (150 ml/$\frac{1}{4}$ pint) fruit juice 2 slices toast with low fat spread and honey or jam
Snack:	2 slices wholemeal bread with 50 g (2 oz) tuna *or* cottage cheese 2 apples (or other fruit)
Lunch:	225 g (8 oz) baked potato with low fat spread 175 g (6 oz) baked beans 1 low fat yoghurt 1 orange (or other fruit)
Snack:	1 bagel with low fat spread
Dinner:	75 g (3 oz) pasta (uncooked weight) 1 tbsp olive oil 175 g (6 oz) white fish *or* cooked lentils/beans 225 g (8 oz) vegetables or salad approx. 4 heaped tbsp fruit crumble 150 ml ($\frac{1}{4}$ pint) custard made with low fat milk
Snack:	1 slice toast with low fat spread 1 banana
	Nutritional information: **Energy: 3080 kcal; carbohydrate: 530 g (64% of kcal);** **fat: 63 g (18% of kcal); protein: 135 g (18% of kcal)**

Snack attack!

Here are some easy to make, high carbohydrate, low fat snacks. They are ideal for women on the run since they can be made in bulk and frozen or stored for several days.

Speedy Apple and Cranberry Muffins

12 servings

265 g (9 oz) self raising flour (white or wholemeal)
75 g (3 oz) brown sugar
1 egg
185 ml (6 fl oz) skimmed milk
3 tbsp melted butter or margarine
80 g (3$\frac{1}{2}$ oz) cranberry sauce
80 g (3$\frac{1}{2}$ oz) apple sauce

- ◆ Mix flour and sugar in a large bowl.
- ◆ Beat egg and stir into flour and sugar.
- ◆ Add milk and melted butter and mix well.
- ◆ Divide mixture into lightly greased muffin tins.
- ◆ Cook at 180°C/350°F/gas mark 4 for 20–25 minutes or until golden brown.

Nutritional information (per muffin):
Energy: 170 kcal; carbohydrate: 30 g (67% of kcal); fat: 5 g (26% of kcal); protein: 3 g (7% of kcal); fibre: 1 g

Cheesy Scones

10 servings

375 g (13 oz) self raising flour (white or wholemeal)
50 g (2 oz) grated, reduced fat cheddar cheese
Grainy mustard
4 tbsp freshly chopped chives (or finely chopped spring onions)
45 g (1½ oz) low fat natural yoghurt
185 ml (6 fl oz) skimmed milk

- ◆ Mix flour, cheese, chives and plenty of black pepper in bowl.
- ◆ Stir in yoghurt, milk and mustard (to taste) to form dough.
- ◆ Knead dough on well floured board and press into a round about 3 cm thick.
- ◆ Cut 5 cm rounds and place on greased baking tray.
- ◆ Brush tops of scones with milk.
- ◆ Bake at 180°C/350°F/gas mark 4 for 12–15 minutes or until brown.

Nutritional information (per scone):
Energy: 150 kcal; carbohydrate: 29 g (75% of kcal); fat: 2 g (9% of kcal); protein; 6 g (16% of kcal); fibre: 1 g

Mix and Match Cake

16 servings

375 g (13 oz) self raising flour (white or wholemeal)
2 eggs
5 tbsp sunflower oil
1–2 tsp vanilla essence
1 tsp salt
200 g (8 oz) brown sugar

200 g (8 oz) raisins
3 large, ripe bananas

+ Mix sugar, eggs, oil, vanilla and salt together.
+ Stir in mashed bananas and raisins and fold in flour.
+ Pour into a well greased baking tin and bake at 180°C/350°F/ gas mark 4 for 40–45 minutes or until cooked.
+ Slice into 16 servings.

Nutritional information (per slice):
Energy: 245 kcal; carbohydrate: 44 g (67% of kcal); fat: 7 g (27% of kcal); protein: 3 g (6% of kcal); fibre: 1 g

For a change, replace the raisins and bananas above with 200 g each of:
– tinned peaches or pineapple (well drained) and grated carrot
– apple sauce and chopped dates
– cranberry sauce and 200 g chopped apricots
– plain or flavoured yoghurt and fresh or frozen strawberries.

Fruit Salad Loaf

12 servings

375 g (13 oz) self raising flour (white or wholemeal)
100 g (4 oz) chopped dried apricots
100 ml (3 fl oz) orange juice
2 apples, grated
1 large, ripe banana
1 egg
150 g (6 oz) sugar
50 g (2 oz) butter

+ Combine sugar, butter, apricots and orange juice in a saucepan.
+ Heat (without boiling) until the sugar has dissolved.
+ Pour into a large bowl and add apple, banana and beaten egg.
+ Sift the flour and fold into the mixture.
+ Pour into a greased baking tin and bake at 180°C/350°F/gas mark 4 for 40–45 minutes or until cooked.

Nutritional information (per slice):
Energy: 220 kcal; carbohydrate: 44 g (75% of kcal); fat: 4 g (18% of kcal); protein: 4 g (7% of kcal); fibre: 2 g

INDEX